# BALANCING YOUR EMOTIONS

Janet —

May He be your balance and keeper!

Gayle Roper

Col. 3:17

I love your work!

# BALANCING YOUR EMOTIONS

## FOR WOMEN WHO WANT CONSISTENCY UNDER STRESS

### GAYLE G. ROPER

Harold Shaw Publishers
Wheaton, Illinois

Train art on page 49 © 1992, Debbie Bryer

ISBN 0-87788-075-1

Cover design by David LaPlaca

**Library of Congress Cataloging-in-Publication Data**

Roper, Gayle G.
    Balancing your emotions : for women who want
consistency under stress / Gayle G. Roper.
        p.    cm.
    ISBN 0-87788-075-1
    1. Emotions—Religious aspects—Christianity. 2. Mental
health—Religious aspects—Christianity. 3. Women,
Christian—Religious life. 4. Adjustment (Psychology)—
Religious aspects—Christianity.
I. Title.
BV4597.3R67  1992
248.8'43—dc20                                           92-30983
                                                            CIP

99  98  97  96  95  94  93  92

10  9  8  7  6  5  4  3  2  1

For Audrey and Cindy,

the lovely and godly young women

my sons have made

my daughters

# CONTENTS

# PART
# ONE

# IDENTIFYING
## THE EMOTIONAL CHAOS
## OF OUR LIVES

We experience "emotional chaos" for a variety of reasons—reasons that are not always clear to us in the midst of daily dilemmas. The first step toward consistency under stress is to identify the specific causes of our emotional ups and downs.

In chapters 1-7 we'll talk about health and its potential effects on our emotions and identify the influence of self-esteem, dreams, and goals upon all we do and are. We'll analyze the confusion that arises when our feelings lead us about by the nose or when we have no patterns around which to build our lives. And we'll discover the difference between real and assumed guilt so that we can break free of the emotional ropes that bind us.

# 1

# EMOTIONAL CHAOS

Junior high school and emotional chaos go together like springtime and baseball. You can't have one without the other.

I remember one specific day in eighth grade. For some reason I had stayed late after school, so I had to walk home alone. I was very distressed at this turn of events. What if someone important saw me walking alone? What if someone unimportant saw me walking alone? What if the people whose houses I had to walk past for a mile and a quarter saw me alone?

My stomach churned and my eyes blurred with tears. I knew a terrible secret was about to be revealed—I was unpopular.

Staring miserably at the sidewalk, I began my journey, not daring to look up. If I didn't see the curtains twitching as I passed the houses, I wouldn't feel the pain as much. If I didn't see the faces staring, I wouldn't hear the whispers: "That poor girl. She's walking by herself, so obviously no one likes her."

Suddenly, a block and a half on my way, out of the corner of my eye, I saw movement on the other side of the street. Cautiously I looked over.

It was Sylvia!

The situation could not have been worse. Sylvia was an upperclassman. She was all that I wasn't: beautiful, popular, a cheerleader. She even had a figure. But worst of all, Sylvia lived on my street. That meant she could see me walking all alone my whole way home. I had never known such humiliation.

It wasn't until years later that it finally dawned on me that Sylvia was alone, too—and who cared?

From my present vantage point of fifty-some years, it's hard to imagine that I felt such emotional pain about such a trivial situation. But I did. It seemed perfectly logical to me that people had nothing better to do than look out their windows and comment on a girl walking home alone. It seemed utterly reasonable that Sylvia's thoughts should focus on me and my shame.

Now I can only shake my head at my foolishness and rejoice that I will never be fourteen again.

## Unexpected Turbulence

But there are times even now when my emotions rise up and surprise me. Let me give an example.

I was taking graduate work in counseling when suddenly I was transferred to a new professor. He observed me with two clients I had already counseled for several weeks. It was his responsibility to meet with me after the sessions and critique my work.

He found fault with me like no one else ever has before or since. He very kindly tore everything I had done to shreds. I remember no positive comments whatsoever.

I responded to his comments in my usual way: I said nothing because I knew I would cry if I opened my mouth. And I knew that tears would destroy what might be left of my academic hopes.

I left his office and drove home, talking to myself the whole way.

"You go to graduate school, kid, you're playing in the big time. If you can't take the heat, the kitchen door is to the rear."

I told my husband Chuck about the situation that evening, basking in his sympathy and trying not to cry. I went to bed and prayed myself to sleep, allowing a few tears in the Lord's presence.

Something awoke me in the middle of the night, and I got up to check on the kids and the cats. I didn't want to waken Chuck, so I didn't turn on the light. Instead I walked full speed into our partially opened bedroom door, cracking my head just over my right eye.

Then I cried. And cried.

Poor Chuck wakened from a deep sleep to find his wife wailing in the doorway.

My emotions had crept up and grabbed me when I wasn't expecting them. Certainly I had hurt my head, but not enough to merit that amount of tears. It was retroactive pain that I was memorializing.

Our emotions are a gift from God, created by him to give our lives richness and meaning. We laugh and cry and love and care and hurt. All of these feelings can deepen us, enrich us, and make us both more thankful to God and more dependent upon him.

Or they can confuse us and warp us and make us forever fourteen.

We all feel occasional emotional chaos as I did. Hurtful things or just plain dumb things happen, and we want to die.

Some of us, however, feel emotional chaos much of the time or at least too much of the time. It's like being permanently in eighth grade. We want to be emotional adults, but somehow we aren't. So what can we do when all we want is peace, yet we experience so much emotional confusion?

*Learning to be consistent in our feelings is a key to emotional peace.*

Proverbs 31:11 and 12 read, "Her husband has *full confidence* in her and lacks nothing of value. She brings him good, not harm, all the days of her life" (emphasis mine).

*Full confidence* or trust. Certainty. Assurance. What a wonderful and desirable personal characteristic. For this man to be so certain about this woman, she must have been consistent. He knew how she would treat him and how she would face difficulties.

Some husbands can be confident that their wives will have snits whenever anything goes wrong. They will be critical, harsh, lazy, temperamental, and/or demanding. But the consistent woman whom a husband or a child or a coworker or a friend can trust brings good into his life, not misery. She brings acceptance, not criticism; love, not pain.

It's not that a consistent woman never cries. It's that she learns how to deal with the feelings that created the tears. It's not that she never hurts. Rather, she learns to handle the feelings that caused the hurt.

And it's not that she never laughs. Her laughter is full—because she has learned to enjoy the feelings that led to the laughter.

Let's look at seven situations that may be preventing us from becoming emotionally consistent: health, wrong goals and expectations, low self-esteem, emotional anarchy, lack of life patterns, assumed guilt, and real guilt.

Then we'll look at some extremely practical, biblical solutions to emotional inconsistency: confession, the old self/new self principle, practice, contentment, and daily commitment.

If you find yourself feeling defeated, guilty, or inadequate, there is help. By the grace of God, emotional consistency is possible.

## *What Do You Think?*

1. What are the main benefits of living with an emotionally consistent individual?

2. Are you such an individual? What are your emotional strengths? What are your emotional weaknesses?

3. Can you think of anyone in your life who has modeled emotional consistency for you? What was the greatest benefit of knowing that person?

4. How about someone who was emotionally inconsistent? What influence did this individual have on you?

5. Read Colossians 3:12-17. What does this passage say to you about emotional consistency? Which of these positive qualities is hardest for you to practice?

# 2

# HEALTH AND HORMONES

I first found out about the profound impact of health on emotions through my husband. For several years Chuck struggled with occasional anxiety that would unexpectedly flare into fear.

The difficulties began when he was in graduate school, and he looked for help from a Christian counselor. The gentleman was very kind and sympathetic but had no particular help or advice except to recommend that Chuck take a job at a smaller company when he finished school because the work pressures might be less.

Chuck followed this advice, but the anxiety still persisted.

I was distressed by the changes this condition had made in my husband. When I first met him, he was almost too cocky. He loved to lead or speak in public. He was tall and slim and very handsome. He handled himself with assurance, and I felt I'd never have to apologize for him or be embarrassed by him. He'd always done well academically and was in a doctoral program when we married.

When this anxiety condition developed, all that self-assurance disappeared. Now it was torture to do something as simple as read a verse in a small group of five or ten. To get up in front of a larger group was beyond him.

When Chuck settled into his job and the pressures of school were gone, the anxiety abated somewhat, but it never went away. For twelve years he struggled, constantly seeking the Lord's help. For twelve years the situation remained the same.

"This must be a spiritual problem," he'd say periodically. "After all, the Bible says, 'Do not be anxious about anything,' and I can't seem to manage that no matter how much I pray about it."

But neither he nor I could see anything in his life that would indicate a spiritual deficiency. Chuck was faithful in his walk with the Lord. He served in our church. He was an excellent husband and father. His speech was always flavored with grace, and he was as consistent and kind in the home as out of it.

I knew that I couldn't see into his secret heart, but actions inevitably flow out of the heart and mind, and there were no actions to indicate a continuing sin problem. In fact, all evidence proved just the opposite: he was a godly man.

Finally Chuck said, "I have to get help for this. We've struggled long enough." And off he went to another counselor.

One of the first things this man did was send Chuck for a full physical including a blood work-up. And—presto, chango—we found the culprit: hypoglycemia.

Low blood-sugar is the hallmark characteristic of hypoglycemia, a measurable abnormality indicative of disease. Sugar, or glucose, provides energy to the body, and when the glucose level in the body isn't high enough to meet the body's needs, hypoglycemia occurs. The brain is particularly subject to insufficient glucose, and when it's deprived, impaired function occurs.

While treatment for hypoglycemia is controversial, Chuck was advised to follow the standard treatment of a high-protein, low-carbohydrate diet eaten in several small meals a day. He was to eat no sugar because the rush of sugar was what caused his body to suppress the glucose in his system.

For a guy who used to eat a package of cookies at a single sitting and bury his cereal in sugar, the new sugar-free diet was torture. But almost immediately he felt so much better that he persevered even until this day, some seventeen years later.

## Not Necessarily Spiritual

The point of this story is that what Chuck was suffering from was not spiritual in any way. It was physical. His low blood-sugar was playing terrible games with his brain and therefore his emotions.

It's important to consider the relationship of health and emotional consistency for two reasons.

1. If health is in some way negatively affecting our emotions, a treatment may be as close as a good doctor.
2. Pinpointing a problem as physical may help us avoid the it-must-be-spiritual trap and its accompanying guilt that Chuck lived with for so many years.

Because of our gender, we women live the bulk of our lives with the effects of bodily functions on emotions. From the time we begin menstruation at approximately 12 years of age until we complete menopause at 55 or so, our monthly cycle affects our disposition and behavior.

## *Menstruation*

I have very clear memories of suffering terrible menstrual cramps each month as a teenager and young woman. I remember the day in high school I stood by the front door waiting for my mother to come take me home because I felt so awful.

One of the guys in my class walked by. "Geez, Gayle," he said. "You look green."

I felt green, and we all know, thanks to Kermit, that it's not easy being green.

I lived at home the first year I taught junior high school, and my father, also a junior-high teacher, gave me some advice.

"Keep control of your class, Gayle," he said. "Don't try to be the kids' friend. In fact, don't smile until Thanksgiving. Take care of your own discipline problems, and don't send them to the office. And whatever you do, don't be one of those women who take off a day every month."

*Uh-oh,* I thought. *I'd better start my period every month on Saturday.*

Besides the physical pain that may be involved, menstruation can also include emotional pain brought on by physical conditions. Premenstrual syndrome (PMS) is the most extreme scenario, and according to Dr. Joe McIlhaney (*1250 Health Care Questions Women Ask,* Baker Book House) 30 to 50 percent of all women have severe enough symptoms to need medication during this time.

The irritability, anger, depression and other psychological changes associated with PMS do not mean that a woman is weak or unstable, or that she has lost touch with God. These changes are the result of physical changes, not a sign of emotional or spiritual weakness. While it is certainly appropriate to pray about these feelings, if they affect a woman's relationships with her husband, her children, or her friends, she should also seek medical help. (p. 143)

## *Post-partum*

Another time when physical changes play heavily on emotions is post-partum. Two to three days after delivery over 80 percent of new mothers feel weepy and lost because of the rapid changes in estrogen and progesterone levels in their bodies. This situation passes rapidly and spontaneously and is nothing more than inconvenient.

However, for one woman in ten, post-partum depression (PPD) sets in, lasting three to four months after delivery. And one in a thousand may experience post-partum psychosis (PPP), a condition so severe the mother may wish to take her baby's life. Again hormones are the major culprit, and the conditions are usually easily treatable.

A woman who wrote to Dear Abby (Philadelphia *Inquirer*, Saturday, March 30, 1991) described her post-partum psychosis. "Following the birth of each of our four children, I went through a period of such severe depression and paranoia that I was a total wreck. . . . It's so difficult to put into words the misery I suffered."

Abby's answer? Information about a support group called Depression After Delivery (Box 1282, Morrisville, PA 19067). Because I was already involved in writing this book and thought the information might be valuable, I contacted the organization to see what I could learn. I received a list of more than 50 names and phone numbers in the Eastern Time Zone, people who would be willing to talk to someone with a PPP problem. There were even names of husbands who will talk to someone who needs time and help. I also received a newsletter and information about a national conference on the subject.

It is interesting to note that while one person in twenty is said to suffer from depression at any given time, 1 out of 4 women of child-bearing age suffers in this manner. Boys and girls suffer depression in the same numbers, and so do adults over fifty, but women in their reproductive years experience depression in much greater numbers than men in the same age group. Much depression, though not all, is physically related.

## *Menopause*

The other stage of life that can cause emotional chaos is menopause. Because many women look at menopause as the beginning of the end, emotions run rampant in the best of circumstances. However, because the sensors in the brain pick up even slight changes in the production of estrogen and progesterone, brain-chemistry is actually altered during this time. Sleep becomes a fond memory, hot flashes and sweats become common, and fuzzy thinking gives cause for great concern.

There has been no significant amount of research done on menopause, but it is estimated that 15 percent of women have no problems with this significant life transition. Fifteen percent more are rendered temporarily dysfunctional, and the vast majority, 70 percent, experience symptoms of varying degrees.

As the body establishes a completely different hormonal pattern, frequently the body is literally at war with itself. Hormonal treatment, especially estrogen, can significantly reduce the symptoms of this warfare, if not completely relieve them. There is controversy about the effects of estrogen on cancers of the uterus and breast, but in most cases it is the preferred treatment for pre- and postmenstrual difficulties. The key is having a physician who acknowledges the very real problems of menopause and deals with them intelligently, tailoring treatment programs to each woman.

I was thrown into abrupt menopause surgically at age 26. I was immediately started on hormone therapy, which I continued for fourteen years before my doctor decided that to continue it further created too much of a cancer risk. I was weaned from the medication and found myself experiencing many of the physical symptoms I'd escaped earlier.

Particularly frustrating to me were the hot flashes that wakened me at 1 A.M., 3 A.M., and 5 A.M. for nights on end. The consistency of these flares of intense body heat fascinated me because I always have trouble being anywhere on time. Yet here was my body regularly overheating on a schedule that my cognitive self never mastered.

In the midst of this struggle I began reading studies on the effect of hormone therapy on osteoporosis, the condition that causes bones to become porous and brittle. Osteoporosis is genetic and strikes one in four women. I pictured my paternal grandmother and grandfather in old age, their bodies shrunk by bone deterioration. On top of the loss of height was my grandmother's dowager's hump, degenerative arthritis, and my father's tendency to calcium deposits at a relatively early age and degenerative arthritis in his last years.

"I want back on the estrogen," I told my doctor. "My chances of trouble from osteoporosis are extremely high, and my chances of cancer are one in many thousands."

Remarkably he had just come to the same decision himself. I began the hormone immediately and will continue it indefinitely. My hot flashes vanished and I felt like myself again, late for everything as usual. Hopefully osteoporosis will not be in my future.

# But Isn't Sin *Sin?*

In considering the emotional effects of physical conditions inherent to women, we come to an interesting and critical crossroads of thought.

What does the Bible have to say about our actions? Doesn't it hold us personally accountable for all our wrong doings? Isn't sin *sin* whatever its origin? Isn't anger always wrong when it attacks and hurts? Isn't speaking to get even or losing our temper always wrong?

Dr. Ed Welch, a licensed psychologist and counselor at the Christian Counseling and Educational Foundation in Laverock, Pennsylvania, writes:

> Even though we are always accountable before God and responsible for sinful behavior, the Bible adds important qualifiers.
>
> Scripture qualifies that, although we are always morally responsible, we are *responsible according to the responses of our hearts*. . . . We are also responsible according to our gifts, talents, abilities, knowledge, and understanding. . . . This puts Christians in the unique position of upholding universal biblical standards while simultaneously being sympathetic to individual differences in abilities. *(Counselor's Guide to the Brain and Its Disorders,* Zondervan Publishing Company, pp. 30-31)

Consider Molly, a woman with severe PMS who has recently become a believer. Molly suffers from an attention deficiency and, though she is very intelligent, barely graduated from high school because of her disability. She has a pattern of screaming and yelling even on good days, but especially at PMS time. When she becomes a shrew, she says she can't help it; it's PMS.

Caryn suffers from PMS also, but she's been a believer since childhood. She has set her heart on living for God, and she deeply loves him. She enjoys studying the Bible and is an accomplished Bible study teacher. When she gets all nervy and mouthy as a result of PMS, she can't decide whether she is justified in excusing herself (after all, it's of physical origin) or guilty of sinning.

When Dr. Welch speaks of responses of the heart and differing abilities, he is referring to things like Molly's spiritual infancy as contrasted with Caryn's long-time relationship with God as well as Molly's learning disability as contrasted with Caryn's enthusiastic studying.

Caryn can rightfully be expected to make a greater effort to control her PMS instead of yielding to it, to make an effort to live in a godly pattern even when it is exceedingly difficult. She can also be expected to understand God's grace and forgiveness when she fails and to seek medical assistance more quickly.

Molly will learn very slowly about personal responsibility and the fact that she should not throw her hands helplessly in the air and say whatever she wants. It will be harder for her to grasp that there is medical treatment available. In the meantime she will continue to be a wild woman on certain days (and God will continue to love her and forgive her).

Brain dysfunction, at least if affected persons are alert and responsive, does not affect the moral capacity of the heart. Therefore those with brain impairments must be treated as image-bearers just like everyone else. To treat them differently would be disrespectful, prejudicial, and unbiblical. (p. 52)

I have always felt it is a special blessing to be a woman. Our minds can be as keen as a man's, but there is usually a sensitivity to other people in women. Whether this sensitivity is innate or cultural is not the issue to me. The issue is that we have this heart-consciousness. Isn't it a tragedy if a treatable health problem limits the use of our greatest asset for serving God?

## SUMMARY

Health problems can have a great impact emotionally.

Just being women forces us to deal with physical issues for the majority of our lives.

PMS, post-partum difficulties, and menopause put special stress on our emotions.

While physical changes in our bodies affect our brains and make emotional consistency difficult, we are always responsible to try to live in godly patterns.

## *What Do You Think?*

1. Have you had or do you presently have a health problem that has affected your emotions? What has helped you cope?

2. Read John 9:1-3, 2 Corinthians 1:3-4, and 2 Corinthians 12:10. What are some of the reasons God allows sickness and weakness?

3. Elizabeth Cady Stanton, an early suffragette who lived very actively into her eighties, wrote in her autobiography that "the heyday of a woman's life is the shady side of fifty . . . " (as quoted by Gail Sheehy in "The Silent Passage: Menopause," *Vanity Fair*, October, 1991). What do you think Mrs. Stanton meant?

# 3

# DREAMS AND DISAPPOINTMENTS

I've been a writer for over twenty years, and I have what I assume to be the same dreams or goals as most other writers.

I dream that people will read something I wrote on purpose instead of by default.

I dream that people will walk into a bookstore and say to the clerk, "Do you have Gayle Roper's latest book?"

I dream that the clerk will say something besides, "Who?"

I dream that the bookstore will actually have a display of my books in one of those little cardboard holders everyone trips over, and the customer won't have to ask about my books because they'll be right there inside the front door for everyone to see.

I dream that editors will fight to publish my books.

I dream that I will be a featured author at the Christian Booksellers Convention, with an autograph booth all my own.

I dream that I will actually make some money with my writing.

But I'm not holding my breath.

Other people have goals and dreams, too, ones that are less selfish or me-oriented than my career dreams. (I am using the words *goals* and *dreams* interchangeably to mean those often unspoken yearning hopes of the heart.)

Ginny volunteered to teach Sunday school full of good will and the warm flush of obeying the Lord's call to service. She wanted to tell those first-grade kids of the grace and glory of God so their young lives would be deeply affected. She wanted to touch them while they were young, while they would listen and learn to love both God and their teacher. She dreamed rosy visions of kids saying, "Thank you, Miss Ginny. You're the best teacher I ever had. You taught me how to love Jesus."

Then she went to class and actually tried to teach.

Joy got married full of hopes and dreams, everyone's good wishes ringing in her ears. She set her goal high: she wanted a wonderful Christian marriage, the kind people would look at and sigh over. She would always be there for her husband and he would always be there for her. People would look at her and Lou and say, "That's what a marriage should be. What a testimony!"

Then she tried to live with this flawed man she had married.

Arlene looked at the tiny, dependent bundle suckling at her breast. Her heart was full of wishes and prayers for this little one: happiness, security, love, success, a strong and personal relationship with Christ. She and this child would not have the problems she and her mother had because she would be smarter about raising him than her mother had been with her. Her son would perceive this and respond positively and lovingly. "Oh, Mom, I love you; you're the best!"

Then the child became two . . . and thirteen . . . and eighteen.

Ginny, Joy, Arlene, and I have set ourselves up for potential failure for two reasons:

1. Our expectations are unrealistic.
2. They cannot be fulfilled without the appropriate actions of others.

# Problem #1—Unrealistic Goals

There is nothing wrong with having high goals. It's wise to hope and plan and try. If we don't attempt, we'll never achieve.

But a little reality should temper our dreams. It can remind us how fantastically high our goals may be and how few people actually breathe the air at that level of accomplishment.

Take my writing goals. When you think about it, how many writers out of the hundreds of thousands practicing the craft actually become known? How many writers can you rattle off as ones you seek out? How many times do you buy a book because of the author as opposed to the topic or the catchy cover?

Ginny may want to make a difference in the lives of her Sunday school charges, but she's forgetting that six-year-olds have an incredibly short attention span and enough undisciplined energy to light New York City.

Joy, who wants the perfect marriage, wants a fine thing. But she's forgetting that two sinners who marry cannot produce a perfect marriage no matter how much they want to.

Arlene wants a wonderful parent-child relationship, a most worthy dream. But to expect no tensions between her and her son, especially when he begins seeking independence as a teenager, is to open herself to great disappointment.

# Problem #2—Dependent Goals

For me to achieve my goals as a writer, I am dependent on an incredible number of people:

- an editor who likes my work and helps me develop it
- a publishing company who's willing to publish it
- an artist who designs an eye-catching cover
- a marketing department that pushes the book
- salesmen who talk it up to store owners
- store owners who stock it—and restock it
- several thousand readers who buy it.

The odds of all these things falling into place are incredibly slim. I know the Lord can work miracles on my behalf, but the truth is that I know many more ordinary writers than famous ones. To put all my eggs in the basket of bestsellerdom is to ask for disappointment.

Ginny, who wants to be the wonderful Sunday school teacher, is dependent on her students for success. And we all know students don't always cooperate.

Joy must depend on her husband for her perfect marriage, and Arlene must depend on her child for that flawless mother/son relationship, and they may not always cooperate. Even when they do cooperate, factors may get in the way of perfection—human frailty, for one thing.

# Realistic Goals

So what's the answer to unrealistic or dependent goals and dreams? No goals or dreams at all?

Certainly not. The answer is to make these dreams and goals secondary and to establish more realistic God-oriented goals.

Instead of wanting to write a bestseller, I must want to be the best writer I can be with God's help. Notice that only God and I come into play in pursuing this goal. Since God is always dependable, my goal is attainable if I am faithful. I still may not sell many books, but I can be *successful*.

Instead of seeking the praise and affection of her students, Ginny should desire to be the best Sunday school teacher she can be by God's enabling. Only she and God are needed to reach this goal, not squirmy six-year-olds. Pleasure in service is still possible.

Joy should want to be the best wife she can be with the aid of God's grace. Again only she and God are involved, and "success" is possible even if Lou doesn't come through.

Arlene should want to be the best mother she can be by God's enabling. Reaching her goal is not dependent on a two-year-old who might stamp his feet and say, "No!" or an eighteen-year-old who may continually break curfew. It's dependent on God's constancy and her faithfulness, and she can know comfort instead of guilt, no matter how things turn out.

If no one publishes my next book, if the six-year-olds riot, if Lou walks out, and if Arlene's son grows up to be a jerk, there will be disappointment and heartbreak, but these feelings don't have to be compounded by a sense of failure. We are not seeking a specific level of achievement but rather to please God with our fragrant offerings of love and obedience. We understand that for the Christian, success is not in accomplishment but in faithfulness. As Paul puts it, "It is the Lord Christ you are serving" (Colossians 3:24).

I began to think deeply about unrealistic and dependent goals when my writing never took off as I had hoped it would. I sold enough to call myself a writer, enough to be encouraged, but never enough to make a reputation for myself.

I called my level of achievement *Mediocre Success* or *Moderate Success*. I originally used the word *mediocre* because I was unhappy with my lack of accomplishment. Not that I viewed my work as mediocre, but I saw my level of achievement as such. *Moderate* is a much better word because it doesn't have the idea of poor quality about it.

I realized that no matter how much I ached to set the world on fire with my prose, I probably would never do so. I had published enough to impress a few friends and my parents, but that was it. I was a moderate success with a desire to be a major one and the sinking realization that I wouldn't make it.

Mid-life crises take root in feelings like mine.

## Whose Goals?

Then the Lord brought this thought to my mind: What is my desire—to reach *my* goals, or to reach God's goals for me?

For God to mold me as he chooses, I may need the hurt of not being what I want to be. I may need the disappointment that makes me dependent, the pain that makes me say, "Father, hold me close." I may need to be limited to moderate success, the very thought of which still makes me gnash my teeth.

And I definitely need to learn to pray with Thomas à Kempis: "Lord, give me the willingness to be obscure."

I also need to remember that Christ accomplished the Father's goal for his life—and he died.

Not achievement but faithfulness.

People came to Jesus and asked him what was the greatest commandment in the Law.

"Love the Lord your God with all your heart and with all your soul and with all your mind and with all your strength," was his reply (Mark 12:30).

It wasn't, "Write a bestseller."

It wasn't, "Model the ultimate parent/child relationship."

It was, "Love God with everything that is in you."

Sometimes people who love the Lord with everything in them do write bestsellers, and some have great success as spouses and parents.

But equally true and less publicized is the fact that many more people who love God deeply and truly never write bestsellers, experience marriages that are stagnant or broken, and rear kids who bring heartache and hurt. These are rarely the people who stand up in church during testimony time. We tend only to hear the "success stories"— successful, that is, in the eyes of society.

Frequently we hear people tell us that we can achieve anything we want if we work hard enough at it. I don't believe this is true. Just ask all the defeated political candidates.

But Paul sets before us the alternative to unrealistic or dependent dreams, the glorious substitute for mediocre success:

"I want to know Christ and the power of his resurrection and the fellowship of sharing in his sufferings, becoming like him in his death" (Philippians 3:10).

The idea of knowing Christ and the power of his resurrection is a bit daunting, but exhilarating. What a wonder to become acquainted with our Savior! What an exciting thing to experience his resurrection power!

But Paul also speaks of "the fellowship of his sufferings" and "becoming like him in his death." Not happy thoughts, but just as much a part of the process of making us godly as the agreeable ideas.

So how do we, in our time and place, fellowship in Christ's sufferings and death? Certainly not like the early Church with its martyrs and physical pain. One of many possible ways is through unfulfilled dreams and goals. There is great pain in laying our hopes aside, especially when we wanted to achieve them in Jesus' name. There is a dying in the loss of fine desires. The heart is torn and the spirit weeps and we lift our arms toward heaven and cry, "Father, help me. I tried. I really tried. What went wrong? No one understands my hurt but you. Only you can even begin to help me handle the disappointment. And you love me anyway!"

In this way we become more dependent and more vulnerable . . . and more godly.

And we take another step in achieving God's goal for us.

## SUMMARY

It is possible to pursue goals that are doomed to failure. We must select realistic goals.

We would do well to avoid goals that depend on others for their accomplishment.

God's goal for us is that we know Christ, his resurrection power, and the sharing of his sufferings.

## What Do You Think?

1. What are your career goals for yourself? Your spouse? Your children? Who is the most ambitious person in your family?

2. How many people are you dependent on to reach your personal goals and dreams? What will you do if they don't cooperate?

3. React to the following statement: "Happiness is too shallow a goal for a Christian." Read and respond to 2 Corinthians 4:8-9, 16.

4. Read Isaiah 38:1-6. What do you think of Hezekiah's prayer? Why did God answer Hezekiah so magnanimously and not other people, probably even some people you know, who asked the same thing?

5. Read Psalm 40:8 and Psalm 143:10. What should be our goal, and how do we achieve it?

# 4

# WORMS OR PRINCES?

---

Let me state up front the thesis of this chapter.

*If you have good self-esteem, that's very nice. If you haven't, God isn't worried. He loves you anyway—and he wants you to live for him anyway.*

The Bible presents a clear picture of who we are as Christians. It's like using an old-fashioned stereopticon where the two different, flat images become a single, three-dimensional picture when we look through the lens. The two views of us humans are both needed if we are to view ourselves properly through the lifegiving lens of God's Word.

### View 1—Unworthy sinners

We are sinners, unworthy of God's love. The phrase from Newton's hymn, "for such a worm as I" is an accurate picture of our standing before a holy God. We may be better than our neighbor, but before the God of the universe, we are full of flaws and rebellion. "You were dead in your transgressions and sins, in which you used to live" (Ephesians 2:1-2).

### *View 2—Beloved children*

We are beloved children of the King, ransomed at a great price. "But God demonstrates his own love for us in this: While we were still sinners, Christ died for us" (Romans 5:8).

Succinctly put, we are sinners saved by grace—nothing more, but, praise God, nothing less. We are wanderers who have been found. We are enemies who have been defeated by grace and taken captive by the King, transformed by his love and forgiveness into his children.

For spiritual health, we need to accept both aspects of our identity—sinner and child. Seeing ourselves only as sinners, offensive to God, denies that Christ's death was sufficient to take care of our sin. But if we see ourselves only as God's blessed children, we will tend to forget the momentous sacrifice Christ made in order to bring us into God's family.

Adjust your stereopticons accordingly.

As believers, the one thing we have in common besides our redemption is our uniqueness. None of us imagines, thinks, speaks the same as another. To me, the most fascinating aspect about God's creation is the amazing variety of the human personality.

When I was a college student, I worked at the New Jersey shore for four summers. One of my favorite pastimes was to sit on a bench on the boardwalk and watch the people parade by. I was never bored because of the variety of things people said and did.

As we look, think, and act differently, so our vision of ourselves varies immensely. Some of us feel confident all the time, some most of the time, some some of the time, and some never. It's the same with the way we view our appearance and our general contribution to society. Some days we just feel more useful than other days. And we rarely have a balanced picture of ourselves.

Why do gifted people think they're terrible? Lovely people think they're ugly? Clever people think they're dumb? Let's look at three influences that form our self-concept.

## Personality Predilection or Predisposition

When my sons were small, I had an interesting conversation with my father.

"How come you never had any great problems with me or my brothers, even when we were teenagers?" I asked, looking for a clue I could carry over into my own child rearing.

He smiled. "It's nothing special your mother and I did," he said. "It's because none of you had a rebellious spirit."

At the time, I was most unsatisfied with Dad's answer because it gave me no handles to grab onto. Now, with my children grown and years of observing other parents and their children, I think Dad was right. It was not in our natures to be troublemakers.

Certainly the nurture/nature debate has been going on for years, and I don't have the answers. But I am convinced that certain traits are genetically coded.

One night when my adopted sons were in high school, we were driving home together. For some reason, Chip, our elder, was feeling complimentary. "Anything good that I accomplish, Mom, is all because of you and Dad."

"That's nice to hear," I said, "but you know it's not true."

"Yes, it is," he insisted.

I shook my head. "You owe a lot to your birth parents, whoever they are," I said. "They passed to you your keen mind and musical ability. All we did was give you a chance to develop them."

"Nope," he said. "It's all you two."

Nature/nurture.

Three children paint pictures. They all do a fine job, each work of art colorful and original. They even look like what they are supposed to represent.

"Let's see your work," says the teacher.

The three hold up their efforts.

The teacher looks carefully and nods. "Very nice," she says, smiling. "You all did a fine job."

Child A beams. *Yes,* she thinks, *I knew it! I did a fine job.*

Child B looks at the teacher and at his picture. *Okay,* he thinks, *if she says it's good, maybe it is. I can live with that.*

Child C looks at the teacher in disbelief. *No!* he thinks. *It's not a good picture. It's a terrible picture! I hate it!*

Any mother of more than one child knows what I'm saying. Any teacher knows. Any Sunday school teacher knows. Some children soak up praise like sponges. Some weigh it carefully and accept it under consideration. Some reject it altogether, no matter how frequently and sincerely it's given.

As intellectual, introverted/extroverted, and rebellious or cooperative spirits are inborn, so is the tendency to see oneself in a certain fashion. Life experiences certainly influence strongly the way any of these tendencies develop, but the predisposition is already present.

## Dissatisfaction or Bitterness

Rarely do our lives turn out the way we as children dreamed they would. One reason is that children tend not to allow reality, sorrow, and tragedy to intrude on their dreams. Rose-colored glasses fit best on small noses.

But real life insists on intruding, and frequently life hurts. Sometimes the hurts are temporary and of lesser consequence (like not making it into a desired club), but sometimes the hurts are huge and life-affecting.

Why God allows his children to suffer such pain is one of the unanswerable questions of life. We know that as God, he could stop the agony, but we also know that frequently he doesn't.

My friend Georgie is the victim of sexual abuse by her grandfather, and she has found that one of her biggest problems in learning to move beyond this memory is anger at God.

"Quite frankly," she told me one night, "I'm so angry at God for not protecting me that at times I don't even want his company."

Some women are angry at God for the families in which they were raised. They might not have had anyone who was physically or sexually abusive in their homes, but the verbal abuse was frequent and extremely damaging. Or the opposite might have been true: no one paid any attention at all.

Some women are bitter over the disappointment their husbands have been. These men have not been as successful, as financially prosperous, as caring, as committed to the Lord as their wives wish.

Some women are very upset with their looks and at root think God should have done a better job. More bosom, less thigh, a smaller nose, fewer freckles—these are large issues to some people.

Some single women are angry at God for not sending along a fine man to marry. They wish to be a wife and resent God's not arranging things for them. After all, he did it for friends who were no more deserving than they, maybe less.

Whatever the cause of this root of bitterness that strangles the flower of love for God, its end result—among other things—is a poor self-image.

## Believing Our Critics

Many of us have long heard messages from the criticizers, the fault-finders, the self-appointed humiliators. Some of them are very outspoken; some are subtle. All of them cause pain.

The interesting thing is that even though we may have several encouragers urging us on to great things and only one critic, we believe the critic. We may recognize that this person has a negative spirit. We may understand that she is flawed. But for some reason, we still believe her.

This tendency is especially strong when a woman has grown up with a critical mother or father or has married a critical man. The constant drip, drip, drip of the fault-finding wears down even the most ebullient spirit and creates self-doubt.

"All I want is for my mother to say just once that I did a fine job!" said Jane with tears in her eyes. "Just once."

It was painful for me to tell her that this hope would probably never be fulfilled no matter how much she longed for it.

"But she's my mother." Pain filled Jane's face. "She's supposed to encourage me. Maybe if she believed in me, I'd believe in me." Jane was fifty-five, her mother seventy-eight.

If you have a predisposition toward feeling bad about yourself, if you're angry at God about some detail of your life, or if you've suffered the demoralization of a critic, it's okay.

No, it's not okay that you were hurt. The inflicting of such pain is never acceptable. You certainly can't be faulted for feeling the pain. God isn't surprised that you don't feel good about yourself, that you feel insecure or dumb.

God does not require us to feel good about ourselves, rather he asks us to have confidence in him. He doesn't ask us to "find" ourselves. In fact, he asks just the opposite. We are to lose ourselves in Christ.

But we have this treasure in jars of clay to show that this all-surpassing power is from God and not from us. *2 Corinthians 4:7*

Jars of clay.

When we became believers, God could have changed us from jars of clay to lovely golden vessels or silver urns or beautiful enamelware chalices, but he didn't. He allowed us to remain clay pots, dinged, imperfect, unlovely, common.

Why did he not make us into glorious creations? Because he wants it to be very clear that any power we exhibit to accomplish anything comes from him as a gift of grace. Not only that, but he wants us to *grow* into beautiful, glorious people. As babies don't—*poof!*—become adults, spiritual growth isn't like a magic spell cast upon us. God's plan has always included growth. When we grow, we learn; as we learn, we *become*.

When a clay pot learns to believe God when he says he loves her, that's God at work.

When a clay pot comes to terms with anger at God and allows God to be God, that's God at work.

When a clay pot learns to believe God instead of the flawed people in her life, that's God at work.

Clay pots could never accomplish feats of that magnitude on their own. They are too human.

The apostle Paul had some sort of a "thorn in the flesh." What it was is uncertain, but we know Paul asked God to remove it. And we know God did not.

Three times I pleaded with the Lord to take it away from me. But he said to me, "My grace is sufficient for you, for my power is made perfect in weakness." Therefore I will boast all the more gladly about my weaknesses, so that Christ's power may rest on me. *2 Corinthians 12:8-9*

A poor view of self may be your "thorn in the spirit." If so, you have the great opportunity to see God prove himself to you. As he was Paul's sufficiency, so he will be yours.

When I was a teenager in that quagmire of negative emotions, I found a verse that helped me see myself as God sees me. It's a verse in Jesus's prayer just before he went to the cross. He is talking with the Father about the believers who are going to come in the future, believers like you and me.

"May [these future believers] be brought to complete unity to let the world know that you sent me and have loved them even as you have loved me," Christ said (John 17:23).

"Wait a minute," I said. "Let's read that again!"

I read the verse again and it still said the same thing. It said that God loved me *even as he loved Jesus*.

I knew all the songs and all the verses that said God loved me, but suddenly it hit me that God loved me with the same kind of love with which he loved his Son! He didn't just love me; he *loved* me!

And he *loves* you, too, with your poor self-image, your anger, your heart full of hurt from your critics.

If I were speaking at a women's group, at this point I would get out a decorative basket about one foot by one foot, some Spanish moss, and a bunch of small plants. I'd take the plants, some with upright foliage, some with drooping grace, one or two with flowers, and place them one at a time in the basket. I'd put the tall ones in the back, the tumbling ones at the front to cascade over the edge of the basket, the ones with blooms where their color would show to advantage.

I would say that each plant is like a woman, different, unique, and attractive in its own way. I would remind the women that none of the plants, like none of the women, is perfect. Some of them have bare spots, some have grown too much on one side of their pot, and some tend to be either a bit too unpretentious or a bit too flamboyant. But they are all special and all necessary to make my garden.

I'd finish by draping the Spanish moss like God's grace around the pots, covering the rough edges and empty spots, and I'd say, "Be the plant God has meant you to be, living the choices he has made for you without bitterness and for his glory."

## SUMMARY

We Christians are sinners saved by grace—and beloved children of the King.

Personality predilection or predisposition may be one reason we see ourselves as we do.

Dissatisfaction and bitterness with the life we have been given cause many of us to see ourselves incorrectly.

Believing what flawed people tell us instead of believing the Bible's view of us causes self-esteem problems.

Being a "jar of clay" gives God ample opportunity to prove himself to us in our weaknesses.

# What Do You Think?

1. What do the following verses say about God's perception of you?

   a. Psalm 139; Luke 12:6-7

   b. Colossians 1:13-14; Psalm 32:1-2

   c. Ephesians 2:10; 1 Corinthians 1:26-29

   d. Isaiah 43:1-3a; Hebrews 13:5-6

   e. 1 Corinthians 12:11, 18; Romans 12:5-6

f. John 12:24-25; Romans 12:1

2. Who knows best what your worth is: your parents? your spouse? yourself? God? Whom will you choose to believe?

# 5

# FLUTTERING HEARTS OR RATIONAL RESPONSES?

---

Which of the following sentences exemplifies the meaning of the verb *feel?*

I feel the president is doing a good job in the day-to-day running of the country.

Or, I feel so good when my two-year-old climbs into my lap, hugs me, and says, "I love you, Mommy."

Or, I feel so excited about the way the Lord is blessing our church. I feel we can make a difference in the lives of the people in our community. I feel God will bless us even more as we rely on him. I feel overwhelmed by all that is happening here.

According to Webster, there are two meanings for *feel*, and all the uses above are acceptable.

The most common definition has to do with our emotions and traces its root to Old English verbs meaning to stroke and to flutter, even to an old German noun meaning

butterfly. *Feel* used this way has to do with internal responses, fluttering hearts and quivering bowels.

The second meaning has to do with thinking, as in feeling the weight of an argument. It has to do with intellect
and argument and rationale.

This distinction is important to keep in mind when we
"think of (ourselves) with sober judgment" (Romans 12:3).
When we say, "I feel . . . " do we mean that we think
something, that we've used contemplation or logic or
reason to come to a conclusion? Or do we mean that our
emotions are telling us something, that we just know it
inside?

Generally speaking, our emotional feelings are reactive,
like two chemicals put together. Something happens or
someone speaks, and we feel. We respond. We retaliate. We
go with our gut.

In contrast, our thought feelings may be proactive, which
means we take the initiative or lead. We analyze things,
think about things, reach conclusions and take action.

Emotions leave us at the mercy of others and ourselves.
Thoughts allow us to be in control.

For the sake of simplicity and clarity, I will refer
throughout this chapter to *thoughts* and *emotions*, rather
than to *feelings*, which is the broader category.

Several years ago in a fit of pique over some act of discipline, one of our kids looked my husband Chuck in the eye
and said, "I hate you."

Chuck was deeply hurt. I still remember finding him
sitting on the edge of our bed looking like he'd been told
that tomorrow he'd become Job.

"He said he hated me," Chuck said.

I tried not to smile too broadly, but I couldn't get too
distressed. I'd already heard that line a couple of times
myself.

"All kids say that," I said. "It's nothing to get upset about."

Chuck just shook his head. It was more than he could fathom that a son he loved and had poured all that time and energy into could say such a thing.

"What did you say back?" I asked.

"I told him that I loved him anyway."

I patted his shoulder. "Good for you. That's what all the books recommend."

"All the books?"

"On raising children," I said. "I told you it's a common thing for kids to say. I first heard it when I refused to let one of the guys have his way when he was about three."

Chuck looked up from his contemplation of the rug. "Didn't it make you feel just terrible?"

I shook my head. "Not really. I expected it to happen sometime. I was ready for it. After I told him I loved him and always would no matter how he felt, I told him that I expected him to say he was sorry because no one should speak to another person that way, especially a kid to his mother."

There was a knock on our door. It was our son looking miserable.

"I'm sorry, Dad," he said. "And I didn't mean it."

Emotions made Chuck reactive to the unkind words of an angry child. But thought allowed me to be proactive, prepared, above the soggy morass of gut response.

## Emotions Are Good

Not that emotions are bad. They most certainly are not. Life would be pretty bland without them.

Recently our church moved into a new sanctuary. Chip and his musical compatriots Tom and Gary wrote a song for the occasion. On dedication morning I was filled with all kinds of wonderful emotions as I listened to Chip, his wife Audrey, Tom, and Gary sing their song.

"I saw you smiling," Chip said later. "It seemed to me that there was this aura of motherly pride shining all around you."

I wouldn't trade those emotions—those *feelings*—for anything.

Nor the emotions when I hear those magic words, "Grandmom! Grandmom!" and see three-year-old Ashley race toward me.

Nor the emotions when Chuck says, "God couldn't have given me a wife more suited to me than you."

I think God gave us emotions for many reasons, but three are worth noting:

- to warn us of danger and potential hurt, as in the fear we feel when we see a speeding car
- to enable us to enjoy the good times and the good things, as in listening to Chip and Audrey's singing
- to bind us to people and causes, as in loving my sons when they were rebellious teenagers.

## Balancing Emotion and Thought

God also had several things in mind when he gave us the ability to think:

- to enable us to develop godly strategies to deal with our situations, as in planning how to deal with a tricky marriage
- to help us grow to the place where we are willing to implement these strategies, as in beginning to build

46

an open relationship with a mother-in-law despite her
criticism

• to enable us to remain committed to our strategies
and relationships even after the emotion has cooled or
gone, as in continuing to do our best on the job after
it's become dull.

What we need is a balance between thought and emotion. If we operate primarily out of thought, we become
cold, calculating, uninteresting. If emotions rule, we're easily swayed, easily led, and life becomes chaotic.

> Then Jesus went with his disciples to a place called Gethsemane, and he said to them, "Sit here while I go over
> there and pray." He took Peter and the two sons of
> Zebedee along with him, and he began to be sorrowful
> and troubled. Then he said to them, "My soul is overwhelmed with sorrow to the point of death. Stay here
> and keep watch with me."
> Going a little farther, he fell with his face to the ground
> and prayed, "My Father, if it is possible, may this cup be
> taken from me. Yet not as I will, but as you will." *Matthew
> 26:36-39*

In this passage we see Jesus feeling deep emotions. He's
sorrowful, troubled, and overwhelmed. Mark says he was
"deeply distressed and troubled," and Luke says his sweat
was like drops of blood. Such a reaction to the Cross is
understandable because Christ knew exactly what he was
going to go through physically, emotionally, and spiritually.

But (and it's a big but) Jesus made a thoughtful, controlled, proactive choice in the midst of his emotions. He
chose to do the will of God. "Yet not as I will, but as you will."

47

There are times when all of us must make choices concerning situations that are loaded with emotional baggage. Our hearts pull one way and our minds pull another. We can't satisfy both. We have to decide, like Christ, whether we'll do what's right, what's best, or merely what we feel like doing.

Take the situation with a girl we'll call Judy. She not only goes to your church but lives just two blocks over, and she's having a rough pregnancy. As a result she's having a hard time caring for her three-year-old twins, Jessi and Jeremiah. It would be easy each afternoon to have the twins over to play with your own three-year-old, Emily, and then put them all down for naps. That way Judy could rest for a while without worry.

However Judy is a critical hypocrite, and you usually just stay out of her way. Taking on the twins will open you to her sharp tongue and her superior attitude. You know that if she's not telling you how you should be raising your kids or caring for hers, she'll be telling you what's wrong with the pastor or your Sunday school teacher or the neighbor across the street. Her fault-finding will activate your own tendency in this area, and you'll become dissatisfied with everything and everyone. And you hate yourself when you're like that!

But the Bible says we're to serve one another and help each other and love one another.

So it's emotions versus thought. It's "I can't get involved with her! She makes me crazy!" against "Let us do good to all people, especially to those who belong to the family of believers" (Galatians 6:10).

Imagine a train made up of three cars: the engine, the coal car, and the caboose. We will label the coal car FAITH, since our faith is where we get the energy and drive to live godly lives. The other two labels we have are THOUGHT and EMOTIONS.

THOUGHT should be the engine on our life's train. It will lead us, transforming the godly energy of our FAITH into the power to move forward for God. EMOTIONS will then be the caboose, definitely a part of the train, but not the part that leads.

This choice allows us

- to be proactive
- to make choices based on what the Bible teaches
- to avoid "shooting from the hip"

Let's go back to critical Judy and her twins. You feel like you don't want to get involved. But you realize that, based on the Word of God, you should get involved.

If EMOTIONS are your life's engine, you will opt out of this opportunity to minister.

If THOUGHT is propelling you forward for Christ, you will care for the twins and ask God's protection from Judy's negative thinking.

But, you ask, doesn't doing what I don't want to do make me a hypocrite? Doesn't it make me as wrong in one way as Judy is in another?

The answer to this question lies in our motivation. Do we help Judy to show everyone what wonderful people we are? To prove to everyone what fine Christians we are? Or are we caring for Jessi and Jeremiah out of obedience to God?

If our motivation is obedience, we are not hypocrites. We are cooperating with God and his purposes. We are obedient daughters.

Let's conduct an experiment. Turn to Ephesians 4. In this passage we find that Paul gets very practical, offering many keys for everyday Christian living:

- live a life worthy of your calling (v. 1)
- be humble, gentle, patient, bearing with one another (v. 2)
- make every effort to keep unity (v. 3)
- speak the truth in love (v. 15)
- live no longer as the Gentiles (v. 17)
- put off your old self (v. 22)
- change your way of thinking (v. 23)
- put on the new self (v. 24)
- put off falsehood and speak truth (v. 25)
- don't sin in your anger (v. 26)
- don't steal but work (v. 28)
- don't say unwholesome words but encouraging ones (v. 29)
- don't grieve the Holy Spirit (v. 30)
- get rid of anger, and be kind and forgiving (vv. 31-32)

If we wanted to list more of these instructions, we would find at least 37 additional ones in the next two chapters. If we look at all these commands (and all the others of Scripture), we would find one interesting thing: nowhere does it say we are to obey if we want to, if we feel like it. It simply says, "Do it!"

Doing it takes thought, not emotions.

## Two Scenarios

How does this idea work out in living? Below are two scenarios that a lonely person might experience. In one example the lonely person yields to her emotions. In the other she thinks and then acts.

1.  Helen is sad and distressed because there are no people in her life who care about her. She wants to pull the covers over her head and cry. In fact, frequently she does. She hates her life, and she wishes someone would come along who would be willing to be a friend, preferably a man. She doesn't know what she'd do without the TV, because without Murphy and Erkel and Balki, she'd truly be alone. God has let her down big time.

2.  Patti is sad and distressed because there are no people in her life who care about her. But because she's read in the Bible that God will never leave her or forsake her, she asks God to fill her with a sense of his presence. She's heard that he's like a friend who sticks closer than a brother, so she's decided to spend time with this Friend on a regular basis. She realizes that even though no one is encouraging her, God still asks her to encourage others, so she asks the pastor where she can help at church. She's still alone most of the time, but the overwhelming feeling of abandonment has lifted. She knows God cares.

Sometimes what we know in our heads must override what we feel in our guts. Notice that Patti didn't feel better before she acted on what she *knew* to be God's will. She had to act thoughtfully even while she felt miserable.

In an era of fast pain-relief medicines, most of us don't understand a concept like this. We want to feel better *now* and will do almost anything to that end. But Christ requires a little more from us, because of the resources we are given through the Holy Spirit. We really can give to others when we feel empty ourselves. We can think through our problems and act in faith when our emotions are still in turmoil. These are not easy tasks. But they are more than possible with God's strength.

My friend Susie is a woman with a heart for God. She is also aware that she is subject to making choices by her emotions, quickly and strongly.

"I've learned I must take time to think," she says. "Sometimes it's as if I pick up my emotions, put them in a chair and leave the room. Then I can pray and hear God."

## SUMMARY

Emotions tend to be reactive while thoughts are proactive.

God created both thought and emotion, and we are most healthy with both in our lives.

If emotions control our lives, we do what we want to do instead of what we ought.

If thoughts control our lives, we are better able to choose well.

## *What Do You Think?*

1. When you look honestly at yourself, do you struggle against domination by your emotions?

2. When you make choices on how to deal with your husband and children, do you react to the situation of the moment, or have you thought about how you will behave ahead of time? (If you are in a group study, share instances when thinking and praying ahead of time made a difference.)

3. Read 2 Peter 3:1-2. Why does Peter write to his readers? How does he encourage the use of thought?

4. Read Philippians 4:6-9. What is Paul's suggested pattern for controlling your life and emotions? On several 3x5 cards write some things that to you are pure and noble and lovely. If negative thoughts are a problem, carry these cards with you and refer to them when you feel yourself slipping into negative patterns.

5. Read Colossians 3:1-2. How does Paul here suggest we keep control of our emotions and our thoughts?

# 6

# PATTERNS OF LIVING

Did you know that women at home with little children, the unemployed, retirees, and ministers share a common problem?

All are subject to depression brought on by lack of a schedule or pattern in their lives. Either no one tells them what to do and when to do it, or if they set an agenda, it often doesn't get followed. Interruptions, crises both small and large, and the demands of other people prevent schedule-keeping.

Any mother can recount tales of day after day when she accomplished nothing she had planned. The baby got sick and took all her energy, both night and day. She inherited her neighbor's three preschoolers when the neighbor was sequestered on jury duty. Her teenagers had to be carted all over the map to their various activities—and these teens apparently had taken a pledge never to belong to the same organizations.

There are times when all of us could pull our hair and gnash our teeth—if we but had the energy. It's then we realize that there's something wonderful about order and planning: they make us think we have some control over our lives.

The major reason we function best in orderly situations is because we are made in the image of One who plans. From creation to the Law, from salvation to the Second Coming, we see a God of order at work.

The plans of the Lord stand firm forever,
the purposes of his heart through all generations.
*Psalm 33:11*

When God established this world, he had a certain goal in mind: the salvation of those who believe in him. Everything he has done for us reveals this priority.

For us to have effective patterns, we too have to establish priorities and decide what we hope to accomplish. Then we plan toward that end. Let's look at three areas of our lives and see how planning works.

## Patterns for Our Spiritual Lives

I have set the Lord always before me.
Because he is at my right hand,
I will not be shaken.
*Psalm 16:8*

"I have set the Lord before me" means that we place him as a counterbalance against the stress, pressure, tension, and chaos of the world. He will keep the scales of our lives stable and prevent us from being overwhelmed and defeated.

Obviously some of the most effective ways of setting God always before us are to worship regularly, to serve in his name, and to spend time with him regularly and often, reading his Word and talking to him.

Several years ago a woman spoke to our church's Women's Fellowship on the topic of prayer. She had with her a large looseleaf notebook.

"I have four small children at home," she said. "I simply can't find the time I'd like for my devotions every day. I know, though, that I need to spend time with God. That's why I developed this prayer notebook. Every morning I write down five requests. I leave the book open on the kitchen counter, and every time I look at it, I pray for the requests."

She held up the book, flipped through the pages, and I was fascinated. She had in her hands a record of her prayers! If I had been asked, I'd have had to admit that I couldn't even remember what I prayed for yesterday, let alone last week or last year.

"Notice the checkmarks and notations on the various pages," the woman said. "They are answers to my prayers. Periodically I go back through the book and write in God's answers."

Now I was really fascinated. She not only had a record of her prayers, but of God's answers! For all I knew, God was answering my prayers, too, but I was too disorganized to realize it.

I determined then and there to start my own notebook. I wanted to see God at work!

I went to the store the first thing the next day and got a binder and paper. I came home and wrote five requests, and I prayed for them off and on all day. I wrote five requests the next day and the next and the next and within a week's time made a startling discovery. I disliked this pattern! I felt it stymied my prayer life rather than enhanced it.

*Maybe*, I thought, *I should write ten requests. I don't have as many kids as she does, so I can pray longer.*

I disliked writing ten requests every day twice as much as I disliked writing five.

*Lord*, I prayed, *I want to see you at work, but I need a pattern that will do for me. Help me!*

I decided that since it was the daily writing that bothered me most, I'd write all my requests down at one sitting. That way I'd be all set. I began writing and the list began growing and I became weary before I'd even prayed a word. There was no way I could pray for all these things every day.

*Lord, help!*

*Divide them up*, I thought. *I can divide them up!*

And so I stumbled onto the pattern I have followed for many years. I got 3x5 cards, one for each weekday. I divided my huge prayer list topically, taking one category a day. Monday I set aside for anything connected with my writing. Tuesday was for my extended family. Wednesday was for friends. Thursday was for missionaries. Friday was for our church and church family. Saturday and Sunday were for whatever was on my heart.

Of course, I pray for Chuck, my sons and daughters-in-law and my granddaughter daily. I also note crisis requests or compelling needs of family and friends in the upper margin of my cards for frequent prayer.

When the Iron Curtain parted, I felt a personal delight because I had been praying for the unknown believers in Warsaw Pact countries, all the Olgas and Sergeis and Vladimirs. But I know I would have forgotten to pray for them if I hadn't written down "believers in Iron Curtain countries" on my cards.

The interesting thing about my prayer pattern is that it may or may not work for you. You may like the notebook idea of the Women's Fellowship speaker. Or you may have a totally different prayer method that works well for you.

That's the catch about patterns. One pattern doesn't accommodate all believers.

One of the things I appreciate most about the Bible is that it doesn't tell us how to do things. It teaches us principles and priorities (like setting God's way always before us), but God in his great wisdom lets us search out our own patterns to fulfill these principles. He allows us to decide what best fits us, our personalities, and our circumstances.

## Patterns for Our Family Lives

Family living is another area of our lives greatly enhanced when we develop workable patterns as both spouse and parent.

Cherry married an engineer who is also an artist. One of the things she liked most about Randall was his sensitive, creative side. It saddened her when, a few years after their marriage and the births of their children, he stopped painting.

"I don't need to paint," he said. "I'm happy with you and the kids. Don't worry."

One summer Cherry had to go to Florida unexpectedly because of the sudden illness of her mother. She took the kids along and was gone almost a month. When she returned, she found her husband painting up a storm.

"It's the solitude," Cherry said, excited about solving the puzzle. "You need solitude to replenish the inner wells of your creativity!"

From that point on, Cherry and the kids went to visit her parents for two weeks each year while her husband stayed home and continued going to work. He also sat by streams and stared, walked alone in the woods, and spent time reveling in silence. And he gathered enough energy to keep his elusive creative streak alive all year.

Cherry told me this story and then asked my advice.

"Some people at church tell me I shouldn't go away each year. It's not right, they say. I'm not being a submissive wife or even a considerate wife when I leave Randall behind. What do you think?"

"Does Randall mind?" I asked.

She shook her head. "He actually likes it. It's the only time the introvert in him is accommodated. Truthfully, I don't go away for myself or my parents but for him."

"The Bible talks about a good marriage in very broad strokes," I said. "That's so every culture and every couple can obey God. Your pattern is different from most people's, but that doesn't mean it's wrong. The Bible doesn't say that you may never visit your parents without your husband. It does say you should honor him and submit to him and be faithful. The patterns you develop to fulfill those principles are up to the two of you."

Maybe the following illustration will explain more clearly the uniqueness of every marriage.

Take a transparent yellow plastic report cover and draw a bride on it. Take a transparent blue cover and draw the groom. Set the sheets on top of each other, hold them to a light and see what shade of green they make.

Every bride comes to marriage her own special shade of yellow. Every groom is his own special shade of blue. Together they create their own unique green. If they try to imitate others, their color is damaged and their potential beauty is marred. They must be themselves and before God develop their own patterns both individually and as a couple. Then both their personal colors and their united color will shine true and bright.

Parenting calls for creative patterning too. Much thought and prayer are needed to determine what is appropriate for you and your family.

At the risk of losing half my readers, I'm going to make a confession. When my sons were still at home, I rarely asked them to make their beds. The reason? I rarely make mine.

I consider bed-making a truly futile task. You go to all that work in the morning just to mess it up in the evening. How does that fit the principles of good time management? I do want to assure you, though, that I firmly believe in changing the bed linens regularly.

I know there are many women who would never leave the bed unmade, who are appalled at my laxity, who would never let a kid go to school without making his bed first. Bed-making is one way to teach responsibility.

And there we have the principle. We must teach our kids responsibility. The Bible tells us to train our children, but again it doesn't tell us how. For one woman it's beds; for another it's something else.

Each fall we as a family sat around the kitchen table and divided up chores for the coming twelve months. I would come to this little council with a list of possible jobs the boys could do. Chip always chose setting and clearing the table and doing the dishes. Jeff always chose the trash, the newspapers, and emptying the dishwasher. Each Saturday they both had to clean their rooms.

If they did their chores, they got an allowance. If not, no money. They could always earn extra for outside seasonal jobs like mowing the lawn and shoveling snow.

"Why do we have to do these jobs?" they would ask periodically. "It's not fair! Lots of our friends don't have to do stuff like this."

And I'd give my three-point lecture:

1.  You are part of our family unit, and each part must contribute to make it work well.
2.  Adult life demands cooperative, responsible behavior, so you might as well learn now and save yourself trouble later.
3.  God asks us as parents to teach you responsibility, and you'll need it to live a consistent Christian life.

The important thing is not *what* you require of your children but that you require *something* of them. Establish patterns that fit your home and your kids. Then establish your own pattern of both holding the kids accountable and encouraging their less-than-perfect efforts.

## Patterns for Our Personal Lives

We need patterns in our personal lives as much as we need them in our spiritual and family lives. It's so easy to become busy with family, work, and church that we take little or no time to evaluate ourselves.

Do not think of yourself more highly than you ought, but rather think of yourself with sober judgment, in accordance with the measure of faith God has given you. *Romans 12:3*

Each of us has certain gifts, and we need to identify them. There are three criteria for determining a spiritual gift:

1.  It is something you do almost naturally.
2.  You enjoy doing it.
3.  Others respond well when you use it.

When I was in my early thirties, I began reading Jill Briscoe's autobiography, *There's a Snake in My Garden.* I was enjoying it, but I put it aside because of some vague discomfort I couldn't identify at the time. In its place I picked up an early book by Ann Keimel. Shortly I put that down with the same feeling.

I tried to analyze what was bothering me because I admired both these women. Finally I figured it out.

Everyone these two women spoke to became a Christian (or so it seemed). Person after person responded to their invitation to trust Christ. Life after life was changed. What I was feeling was guilt because almost no one I spoke to became a believer. Obviously I was doing something wrong.

I realized, though, that being upset because people were coming to Christ was—to put it mildly—foolish. I thought some more and came to the following conclusion: these two women have the gift of evangelism and I do not. Instead of feeling threatened by them, I needed to rejoice that they are so effective.

Of course I must still share the Lord whenever possible, but I accept the fact that I'll never receive the response they do. And it's all right. I'm not them, and I have my own strengths.

I went back to both books with this new insight and finished them, rejoicing that some are so effective in bringing people to Christ.

As we look honestly and soberly at ourselves and consider how we can avoid emotional chaos, we need to look not only at our gifts, but at the constraints of our specific lives.

How old are our children? Can we do what we want or must we yield to their present needs? We only get one chance with them, and we don't want to mess it up.

Do our husbands travel a lot or are they home every night? Do they help with the children? Are they doers or thinkers? Do they support us readily or do they need to be convinced? Or will they never be convinced?

How much time do we realistically have to use as we choose? After we finish working, taking care of the family, helping with homework, and doing the laundry, do we have time or energy for outside involvements? What responsibilities do we have that no one else can fulfill? What commitments do we have that someone else can do?

It's important to be realistic, not fatalistic, about the limitations of our lives. All of us have people and responsibilities that get in the way of "self-fulfillment." Assess these limiting factors and determine just how truly limiting they are.

Mindy became a Christian after her marriage, and her husband Ed has been skeptical about her new faith. Like many new Christians, Mindy wants to be around other believers. She loves to hear the Bible taught to slake her thirst for the things of God. If she could manage it, she'd be out every night at some Bible study or another while Ed watches their three young children.

But Mindy is realistic about her situation. Even if Ed were a believer, every night out would be much too much. And she understands that it's quite normal for him to want her with him instead of with people he's afraid are slightly wacko.

"I don't want you to go out at nights," Ed says. "I stay home to be with you and the kids. I want you to do the same thing."

So Mindy has adapted her schedule and her desires to meet her limitations. Sunday morning services and Wednesday morning Bible study give her opportunities to learn the Word, and she avoids offending her husband.

Creativity and accommodation are key words in finding solutions to the strictures of our lives. We're adults for a long time, and we don't need to experience everything today.

## SUMMARY

Patterns for living are important because we are created in the image of One who plans.

In our spiritual lives we want to "set the Lord always before us" in a pattern that enables us to grow in him.

In our family lives we need to develop patterns of relating to our spouses and teaching responsibility to our children.

In our personal lives we must consider both our gifts and the limitations of our circumstances.

## *What Do You Think?*

1. What do the following verses tell us about order and patterns?

John 2:4

Galatians 4:4

1 Corinthians 14:40

Philippians 4:9

2. To establish valid patterns, we must know our priorities. As you answer the following question, it will tell you much about your priorities. *When you die and people look back on your life, what do you want to leave as your legacy?*

3. Merely thinking up patterns isn't enough. Read John 17:4 and 2 Timothy 4:7. What else is required?

# 7

# THE GUILT TRAP

When I was growing up, my mother told me, "Never marry a man who comes home for lunch."

I figured she knew what she was talking about because my father was everything from a self-employed piano tuner to a public school teacher. When he taught and when, during World War II, he worked at New York Shipyard (located in Gloucester, New Jersey, near Philadelphia), he didn't eat lunch at home. When he sold real estate and tuned pianos, he did.

I didn't decide to marry Chuck because of his future lunch plans, but I admit I like the fact that even though his work place is only ten minutes away, he doesn't come home until dinner. I have the freedom to plan my own day without having to consider his sandwich and chips.

So it was a surprise recently when I was working in my office at home and heard our garage door go up. I glanced at the clock. It was just past noon.

Chuck rushed in. "If I hurry," he said, "I'll have forty minutes to work on the lawn. I want to finish raking so I can put the crab-grass killer on this evening. I need to do it right away because it's supposed to rain for the next couple of days."

I nodded and went back to my work. Within our mutually agreed-upon job descriptions, the lawn is Chuck's responsibility. Mine's the garden, and it doesn't need crab-grass killer.

"Of course you can help me," he said graciously. "Just get a rake."

Help him? I can't help him. Procrastinator that I am, I'm too far behind in my own work. I've got to finish planning the writers' conference brochure. I've got to write some more on the book fast nearing deadline.

"But then," he said, glancing at my lighted computer screen, "maybe you're too busy to help me." And he got the leaf eater and went to work.

*Guilt, I thought. I'm doomed to guilt! If I don't help him, I'll feel terrible, and if I do help him, I'll feel terrible. My choice is: which option makes me feel less guilty?*

My mother was right!

For the sake of accuracy it's important to realize that there are two broad categories of guilt—real guilt and assumed guilt. Realizing which category a particular difficulty falls into helps us determine what to do in order to control the situation.

Real guilt as I'm defining it is our accountability before God for failing to keep his standards. The word *guilt* derives from an Old English word *gylt*, meaning sin. *Real guilt* exists when we commit an act against God or people that doesn't meet God's criteria of holiness.

One doesn't have to feel sorry for this wrongdoing to be guilty. A murderer may feel no contrition for his crime, but he is still guilty. Guilty is something we are, not something we feel.

*Assumed guilt* as I'm defining it has to do with regret, remorse, or failure. It is a matter of misjudgment and accident rather than sin. What I was feeling when I didn't want to rake with Chuck was assumed guilt. Sin wasn't an issue (though it could have been if anger and resentment and selfishness had been involved). It was an issue of time, an issue of not being able to do it all, a regret that I was either going to let Chuck down or not get my work finished.

The wonderful thing is that Christ is there for us whether we are struggling with real or assumed guilt. He is both the Savior of sinners and the Bearer of burdens.

(I did go outside and ask Chuck what he wanted me to do, not because I wanted to rake, but because I felt serving him in this manner was important. He in his turn sent me back inside, apologizing for putting me on the spot. "Go do your work," he said. "That's your first priority right now.")

## Real Guilt

If our own honesty won't admit that we are guilty of failing to meet God's standards, then the Bible will thunder this truth. "All have sinned" (Romans 3:23) leaves no room for escaping God's opinion. All have sinned, even the nice guys and the good girls.

Since the criterion is God's holiness, it's not hard to see why we have all fallen short, way short, and why we are guilty whether we feel it or not.

It is because of this very real guilt and its attendant separation from God that Christ became our sacrifice. When we believe in Christ as the Savior who took our sins upon himself when he was crucified, our very real guilt is forgiven. Our position in Christ makes us guiltless in God's eyes.

What a wonderful truth! We cannot be spiritually condemned as guilty because in Christ we are guiltless! God is not our Judge but our Father! "Therefore, there is now no condemnation for those who are in Christ Jesus" (Romans 8:1).

When we are guilty of breaking human laws, punishment is the standard way of dealing with the crime, whether it be a fine, so many years in jail or so many hours of community service. Many times, the acts the state finds reprehensible are the same deeds God holds us accountable for. The difference is that where the state punishes, God through Christ forgives.

While our forgiveness assures us of acceptance by God, we are not exempt from the consequences of sin in our lives. When the Old Testament writers referred to the sins of the parents being visited on the children to the third and fourth generations (Exodus 20:5; Deuteronomy 5:9), what they were referring to was consequences. A dysfunctional family breeds dysfunctional kids, grandkids and even great-grandkids. Logical consequences. Only the power of Christ is strong enough to break these terrible patterns and offer hope.

While salvation and forgiveness make us sinless in one sense, we still do sin. There is a thought in Romans that I frequently pray because I know my tendency to excuse myself and to minimize my guilt. I pray that "sin might become utterly sinful" to me (Romans 7:13). In other words, I want the Holy Spirit to teach me when I am offending God, when I am truly guilty. God may no longer be my Judge, but he is my Father, and as his loving child, I desire to please him.

# Assumed Guilt

## *Failure*

Pat had quite a collection of plants, all given to her when her husband died. Every week she watered them carefully. Every week as she did so, she felt full of guilt.

*How is it,* she'd think, *that I can keep these stupid plants alive, but I couldn't keep Tom alive?*

Finally, distressed and haunted by the emotions the plants caused, she threw them all out.

"I knew what I was feeling was illogical, but I kept thinking I should have been able to do something for Tom, something to make him better or something to bring him back. The plants symbolized my failure."

Failure. How we hate it. We hide it from others. We deny it to ourselves. Often, because of our culture, we assume that failure is an offense against God.

The truth is that many fine Christians fail in business, in school, in relationships. While it is accurate that sin may lead to failure in any of these areas, it is equally true that failure can come where there is no sin. In fact, a desire to do God's will and honor him may be very much in the heart of the person who fails.

When such a failure occurs, some good questions to ask are:

- By whose standards have I failed?
- My family's?
- America's?
- My own?
- God's?

It is very possible that we have disappointed our families and ourselves, but we don't disappoint God by failing. His desire for us is NOT success. It is, as the Westminster Catechism says, that we love him and enjoy him forever. It is that we become like Christ. Our failures do not make us unacceptable to God or make him love us any less—just as our successes do not make us more attractive to him or cause him to love us any more.

God's purposes for us can be reached in failure as well as in success, for failure, like illness or bereavement, can be his tool to develop us and make us more dependent on him. Failure makes us vulnerable and teachable. It may well be one of his greatest gifts to us.

### Remorse, sorrow, and regret

If failure is frequently mistaken as something over which to feel guilt, so are remorse, sorrow, and regret. However it's important to remember that there doesn't need to be an offense against God for these emotions to exist. There need only be a misjudgment or an accident.

When I sneeze, I never sneeze once. My minimum is five, but frequently it's more. At times, I've had a sneezing fit while driving, not a comfortable situation because every time I sneeze, my eyes close involuntarily. If a child ever ran out in front of my car at such a time, I might not even see him.

If such a terrible thing did happen and I hit that child, I would feel overwhelming sorrow and remorse. My whole life would be dramatically and deeply changed by such an accident.

But note, the operative word here is *accident*. Personal sin is not connected to this scenario any more than it was to Pat and the feeling of failure her plants brought. Accidents just "happen" because an unlikely set of circumstances comes together. Just as godly people fail, they have accidents and make misjudgments that bring great pain. And God works through these events just as he does through failure.

Why do I make a distinction between guilt on the one hand, and failure, accidents and remorse on the other? Because I don't want any of us to carry a double burden unnecessarily. If we have not offended God in a particular situation, we don't need to seek his forgiveness concerning it. Rather we need to ask for his strength, his compassion, his ability to repair the irreparable. "Come to me," Jesus said, "all you who are weary and burdened, and I will give you rest" (Matthew 11:28).

## Forgiving ourselves

There is another type of assumed guilt worth noting, and it has to do with confessed sin.

In many of our lives there is a particular sin we committed, often many years ago. This sin is especially reprehensible to us, and we have confessed it so many times we've lost track. Every time we remember it and the pain it caused (and causes) and the distress we felt (and feel), we confess. Our hope is that finally, eventually, we will feel cleansed.

I had such a sin in my life. Every time I thought about it, I'd pray, "Oh, Lord, forgive me! I'm so thankful I don't do this anymore, but I'm so sorry I ever did it. Forgive me!"

One day I realized a specific truth. *The first time I had asked God to forgive this action, he had done so.*

It is not in God's character to play games with us. He doesn't sit up in heaven watching us, making us squirm with guilt. Rather, "If we confess our sins, he is faithful and just and will forgive us our sins and purify us from all unrighteousness" (1 John 1:9).

When I kept asking for forgiveness for the same sin over and over, I was saying that Christ's sacrifice wasn't sufficient for me. What I did all those years ago was too terrible for him to handle. His death atoned for all the sins of all the world except this particular one of mine, and I had to keep pleading with God over it.

Of course I didn't mean to devalue Christ's death by holding on to my assumed guilt, but I was doing so nonetheless.

I also realized about this same time that one of the Enemy's favorite ploys is to accuse believers (Revelation 12:10). He does this by reminding us of our sins and our accidents and making us feel terrible about them. We become embarrassed and guilt ridden, and we turn from God because of this shame. A wedge is driven in our relationship with God, a wedge we help drive by believing our feelings of guilt rather than God's promise of forgiveness.

But how, someone may ask, can I recognize when I am being accused by the Enemy as opposed to when the Holy Spirit is convicting me about something I honestly need to correct?

There are two tests we can apply to make this determination:

1. Have we confessed our sin to God, admitting our guilt and asking his forgiveness? If the answer is yes, then the feelings that persist are accusations.
2. While Satan seeks to drive a wedge between us and God, the Holy Spirit, on the other hand, seeks to reveal our sin to us so that we can restore our damaged relationship with our Father. Satan is divisive; the Holy Spirit is a healer.

Remember my problem with assumed guilt over a long-ago sin? In order to silence the accusatory voice within me, I got down on my knees and prayed, "God, I realize you forgave me years ago, the first time I came to you about this sin. You chose to do that for me even though I didn't deserve it. It is not of you that I still feel guilty over this issue. I want this day to be a watershed in my Christian life, a day I can look to every time I remember this sin, every time the Enemy accuses me. Because of Christ's death and based on the promise of 1 John 1:9, I know I am forgiven and free."

Now whenever I think of this issue, I recite 1 John 1:9 and remember my forgiven state. Instead of regret and embarrassment, I rejoice in the graciousness of a God who doesn't keep accounts against us.

## SUMMARY

There are two types of guilt, real and assumed.

Real guilt is our culpability for failing to meet God's standards. Guilty is something we are, not something we feel.

Failure, remorse and Satan's accusatory voice may be mistaken for real guilt when in fact they are assumed guilt.

Jesus is both the Forgiver of sins and the Bearer of burdens.

## *What Do You Think?*

1.  Read Psalm 130. What promises are here for those experiencing real guilt?

2.  When we confess our sins, what great gift does God give us?
Psalm 32:5

Colossians 2:13

3.  Scripture urges us to confess or acknowledge more than just our sin. What do these verses tell us?
Romans 10:9

Matthew 10:32

1 John 4:15

2 Corinthians 9:13

4. If we suffer from assumed guilt, from failure or remorse or pain, what do the following verses offer as hope?

Psalm 7:1

Psalm 18:1-3

Psalm 32:7

Psalm 46:1

Isaiah 25:4

1 Peter 5:7

# PART

# TWO

# CONTROLLING
## THE EMOTIONAL CHAOS
## OF OUR LIVES

I've always found it far easier to assess problems, to name them, to tsk-tsk over them, than to correct them. However, just putting a name to a difficulty doesn't reduce it. We may know now what to call our problems, but controlling these areas is as great an issue as it ever was. It's time for specific, practical means of developing emotional consistency.

The concepts we are about to discuss, when applied and accompanied by dependence on God, can make a great difference in the quality of our Christian lives. We are going to examine:

- repentance and confession
- the old self/new self concept
- the need to practice godly living
- the place of contentment
- the absolute necessity of daily commitment

*Lord, teach us what we need to learn, and give us the wisdom and courage to act on this knowledge.*

# 8

# CLEANSING CONFESSION

I grew up in New Jersey, a state where you must be seventeen before you can get your driver's license. For me this was no great hardship in spite of the fact that just across the Delaware River in Pennsylvania sixteen was the magic age.

However the wait of that extra year apparently was difficult for my older brother, an honor student and Student Council president. One day when my parents were out, Chuck couldn't wait any longer.

Yes, Chuck. As a point of confusion, I must tell you that I have eight Charleses in my immediate family. On my side it's my grandfather, father, brother, and nephew. On the Roper side it's my father-in-law, husband, son, and nephew.

The first time my husband, then merely a new boyfriend, came to dinner, there were six people at the table, three of them named Chuck: my father, my brother, and my boyfriend. In the course of the meal, my father Chuck offered the mashed potatoes to my boyfriend Chuck with a smile, saying, "Have some more potatoes, Bob."

Bob was my recently departed old boyfriend.

In the small stillness that always follows mistakes of this kind, Dad cleared his throat. "I called you Bob because there are just too many Chucks around this table." Which scarcely made things better.

Later that evening as I was getting ready for bed, Dad came to my door. "I hope I didn't give that guy the impression I wanted him to disappear with my too-many-Chucks comment," he said. "Really, I think he's the best thing you've brought home yet."

So I decided to keep him.

Anyway, my *brother* Chuck was feeling the restrictions of being too young to drive. One day with Mom and Dad gone in one car and not due back for some time, he took the other car for a little spin. Unfortunately for him, Mom and Dad got back a lot sooner than expected, and they were watching out the window when Chuck drove up out front.

"I never saw anyone go as pale as he did when he saw our car in the driveway," said Mom with a gentle laugh. "Talk about being caught red-handed!"

As I recall the story, no one said anything to Chuck about his little drive for a couple of days. Remember, this is a kid who rarely did anything wrong. My parents decided that stewing in his own guilt was a more effective punishment for him than a lecture or social restrictions or some other quick resolution. It must have worked. He never took the car again.

Guilty. We are all guilty. We are observed in the act by our Father who knows everything, just as my brother was by my parents. To my brother's credit, he never tried to explain or defend himself. He was wrong and he knew it. Incredibly, many of us still try to talk our way out of our actions as if we could convince God that he should have a different set of standards for us.

"Hey, everybody cheats on their taxes. It's not such a bad thing to do. I mean, it's not murder or anything."

"I know you asked me not to say anything, but Janny wanted to know what was wrong. This way she could pray for you, too. But don't worry. I told her not to tell anyone else."

"The cashier gave me a ten instead of a one for change. You know how things have been so tight for me recently. Boy, this is sure my lucky day!"

It is absolutely imperative for emotional health and consistency that we be honest with ourselves and others. The issue is not *whether* we have broken God's standard in a big or little way. The issue is that we *have* broken it, period, and we must acknowledge it.

A few weeks ago our son Jeff was preparing for the opening day of fishing season. He got his rod and reel all ready, and he bought a good supply of worms, which he put in the refrigerator overnight.

Ashley, his three-year-old and the most wonderful little girl in the world, was curious about what was in the worm box. Jeff opened it and showed her the worms crawling around in their dirt.

Ashley got so excited she started dancing. "Oh, Daddy," she said. "You've got sidewalk snakes!"

In truth, no matter what Ashley calls a worm, it's still a worm.

The same way, no matter what we call an action that falls short of God's standard, it's still sin.

I don't think there's any cure for being a worm, but there is a remedy for believers who are entangled in sin, no matter how major, no matter how trivial.

The first part of the cure is repentance; the second is confession.

# Repentance

Repentance is basically changing one's mind, and we can repent of all types of things. We can repent about buying that red and orange dress. We can repent about quitting our jobs. We can repent about our feelings for someone. For the purposes of this book, however, we will use the narrow theological definition of *changing our minds about our sin.*

We need to change our minds about cheating on our income tax, acknowledging it as wrong.

We need to change our minds about passing on privileged information, admitting we broke a trust and betrayed a friend.

We must change our minds about the ten mistakenly given us by the cashier, agreeing that keeping that money was stealing.

Frequently it's sorrow that causes us to acknowledge our wrong behavior. Paul writes about "godly sorrow," the sadness we experience when the Holy Spirit teaches us that we have offended God (2 Corinthians 7:10).

Godly sorrow may cause us to pray, "Oh, God, I feel so awful about what I've done. I can't sleep at night, I can't eat, and all I want to do is cry. It seemed like such a good idea at the time, but I know now it wasn't. It was wrong. Forgive me."

It is also possible for God's kindness to bring us to repentance (Romans 2:4). We do something that offends God, and he still blesses us, still cares for us, still loves us. We are overwhelmed by his kindness.

Then we might pray, "Oh, God, you are so good to me. I am so ashamed of the way I have disobeyed you and hurt you when all you do is love me. Forgive me for my wrong actions."

It's been my observation that we all repent in different ways, some with tears, some dry-eyed, some with upset stomachs, some with improved digestion. It's a matter of temperament and background. The emotion we may or may not feel is not the important thing; the *changing of our minds* to bring our thinking in line with God's is.

## Confession

Repentance and confession are closely related, but there are differences worth noting.

As we can repent of any number of things, so we can confess any number of things. We can confess our real ages when someone tells us we look younger. We can confess that we love someone, either to the loved one or to another. We can confess that we took the last chocolate chip cookie. For our purposes we will use the biblical definition of *saying the same thing as God* or *agreeing with God*.

When we confess our sins, we are agreeing with God that not only are certain behaviors wrong, but we were wrong to do or think them.

We now agree with God that cheating on our income taxes is wrong.

We now say the same thing as God about passing on gossip.

We now agree that keeping the ten was theft.

Repentance and confession are where we must begin if we want to get and keep control of this squiggly, slippery thing called life. We have to examine ourselves and our actions and ask some very hard and possibly painful questions. And we must be scrupulously honest with ourselves. We must ask God to make sin exceedingly sinful to us.

What areas of our lives are out of sync with God's standards and require us to change our minds about them?

What activities and thoughts do we need to confess as wrong?

In other words, where are we failing as Christians to be wholly devoted followers of Christ?

And what are we willing to do about it?

Several years ago I was on a parent-teacher task force at the kids' elementary school. All the other schools in the district had similar panels. Our task was to examine the school, the curriculum, and the school district and then pass on both our concerns and ideas for correcting any weaknesses.

We met several times, and we came up with a list of things that concerned us, things like teacher-student ratios, more reading time, better vocational training for non-college-bound kids. However, we couldn't come up with many practical ideas on how to correct these concerns without spending gobs of money that the district didn't have.

Just as the task force outlined the problems that kept the schools from being all they could, so we have defined problems that may disrupt and limit our lives. But—and it's a very big but—unlike the task force that couldn't correct the problems in public education, we as believers have the wherewithal to correct our life problems. Where the task force had limited resources and limited opportunity to make a difference, we have at our disposal the very power of God in the Person of the Holy Spirit to enable us to see our shortcomings and then change as we need to.

As we've already seen, these changes begin with repentance and confession, but they don't end there. Coming to

God's conclusions does not immediately revamp one's whole life. However, it begins the process.

## SUMMARY

We must acknowledge our problems and our sin if we hope to correct them.

Repentance is changing one's mind about an action or thought.

Confession is agreeing with God about one's action and thoughts.

Repentance and confession are the beginning steps in the process of getting control of our emotions.

## *What Do You Think?*

1. Read Psalm 38. What caused David, that great man of God, to repent? What did he confess? What was the result in his life of harboring sin?

2. If you change your mind and agree with God, what do you expect to happen?

3. Read 1 John 1:9. What does this verse say about the wrong things you have done or the good things you have left undone? What about the things you aren't even aware of?

# 9

# THE PUT OFF/PUT ON PRINCIPLE

Tammy Boatwright woke up Monday morning before the 6:30 alarm rang, a very unusual experience for one who thought bedtime should be between midnight and one and rising between eight and nine. She lay quietly beside Hap, eager for the day to begin.

*Lord,* she thought, *today's going to be such an exciting day! I can't wait to see how you help me.*

For some time now, Tammy has known that she had to do something about her mouthiness. Somewhere, somehow, she had stopped speaking nicely to the people she lived with.

Granted, four sons aged two, four, six, and eight, and a husband who acted like a ten-year-old half the time were enough to make most women sound off. It was a matter of self-preservation.

But she knew she did more than sound off, and she'd never read about self-preservation in the Bible.

"Darren, you're such a bully! Leave your big brother alone. Who do you think you are, you little animal? I ought to give you to the zoo! Those lions would shape you up in no time."

"Carlton, you turn that TV off before I wring your neck! I told you to go to bed, and I mean it! Off, off, off, you terrible kid! What did I ever do to deserve you?"

"Barton, you shut your mouth before I shut it for you! I don't want to hear any complaints! Just once I want you to be a good boy and do what I ask without me having to throw a fit. Come on, surprise me once before I have to visit you in jail. That's where bad kids end up, you know."

"Alvin, you can be so dumb! Look where you're walking, why don't you? You can see, can't you? Your eyes are still in your head, aren't they? There should be plenty of room for them because you obviously have no brain!"

Tammy shivered as she thought of all the nasty things she'd said to her sons. In reality she loved them dearly, but she never sounded like it. It was easier to yell. *Her* mother had always yelled.

"I'll never be like that when I have kids," Tammy had told Hap when they were dating. "I hate the way she talks. I hate the way she always makes me feel. I promise never to speak like that to you or any kids we might have."

Now eight years later she made her mother sound like Cinderella's fairy godmother.

Yesterday in church she had listened to the pastor speak on the tongue. It was James 3:9 and 10 that convinced her she must do something.

"With the tongue we praise our Lord and Father, and with it we curse men, who have been made in God's likeness. Out of the same mouth come praise and cursing. My brothers, this should not be."

"Oh, God," she had prayed. "I've been so wrong! Help me not to speak so unkindly. Help me not to be so mean to my kids and to Hap. Help me not to be like Mom!"

Now she was ready to change. When the alarm went off, she got up right away.

"Are you sick?" asked Hap. "Don't you feel well?"

"I'm fine," Tammy said defensively. "Why do you think I'm sick? Are you saying I look terrible or something?"

"You just got out of bed without complaining and griping. You always make a scene about getting up."

"I don't like mornings," Tammy said stiffly.

Hap sighed. "Tell me about it."

"Look, Mister," spat Tammy, "you're no ray of sunshine at 6:30 yourself."

"Of course not," Hap said. "I live with you."

With that he slammed the shower stall door behind him.

"That's right," she fumed as she put the toothpaste on her toothbrush. "Run out on our discussion."

"Discussion?" he yelled over the sound of rushing water. "Discussion? We haven't had a civil discussion in years!"

"And whose fault is that?" she yelled back.

"Not mine, sweetheart," he said in a tired voice. "Not mine."

"So it's all my fault, huh? Of course! I might have known. Blame it on Tammy. Then your conscience is clear. Well, I'll tell you something, Hap! I'm not going to fight with you anymore." She stamped her foot for emphasis. "I'm turning over a new leaf tomorrow morning!"

Five minutes out of bed and already Tammy has blown her good intentions. How could it have happened when she was so sincere? When she meant so well?

# The Positive Replacement

Tammy experienced disappointment and failure because she grasped only part of the process of godly change in our lives.

Tammy understood the negative part of the equation. She wanted *not* to speak unkindly and combatively. She understood that such speech dishonors God.

However Tammy never thought far enough to develop a positive *replacement* for the negative pattern she wanted to abandon. When she thought only of putting off her nasty speech patterns, she created a hole, a void, a vacuum.

In life as in nature, a vacuum cannot exist. Something will always rush in to fill the empty space. When the crunch comes, what rushes in is our old behavior, our old habits.

When Hap got sharp, Tammy had only a vacuum of good intentions to respond with. Back scurried her old patterns of speech. The known, no matter how much it is hated, will win out over a vacuum every time.

> You were taught, with regard to your former way of life, to put off your old self, which is being corrupted by its deceitful desires; to be made new in the attitude of your minds; and to put on the new self, created to be like God in true righteousness and holiness. *Ephesians 4:22-24*

These verses show us the three-step process we need to follow in order to successfully change our bad habits.

1. We "put off" our old sinful self. In other words, we recognize what's wrong and determine to stop.
2. We "become new in the attitudes of our mind." We learn to think about our area of weakness as Christ thinks about it.

3. We "put on" the new self. We replace our wrong actions and attitudes with godly ones.

The rest of Ephesians 4 explains clearly how we are to act on these steps.

Therefore each of you must put off falsehood and speak truthfully to his neighbor, for we are all members of one body. *Ephesians 4:25*

1. Stop telling lies.
2. Agree with God that lying is wrong and telling the truth is right.
3. Start telling the truth because we are believers and should help each other.

He who has been stealing must steal no longer, but must work, doing something useful with his own hands, that he may have something to share with those in need. *Ephesians 4:28*

1. Put off stealing.
2. Agree with God that stealing is wrong and working is right.
3. Begin working so you'll have a way to share with others.

Do not let any unwholesome talk come out of your mouths, but only what is helpful for building others up according to their needs, that it may benefit those who listen. *Ephesians 4:29*

1. Put off saying things that hurt.

2. Agree with God that speaking nastily is wrong and speaking kindly is right.
3. Put on helpful speech—encouraging speech—in order to build others up.

Get rid of all bitterness, rage and anger, brawling and slander, along with every form of malice. Be kind and compassionate to one another, forgiving each other, just as in Christ God forgave you. *Ephesians 4:31-32*

1. Put off all forms of anger and bitterness.
2. Agree with God that speaking or thinking with animosity is wrong and showing kindness, compassion, and love is right.
3. Put on compassion and forgiveness because in Christ God has forgiven you.

## Godly Thinking

Please note that knowing these three principles doesn't make restructuring our lives a snap! We will talk more in the next chapter about the need to persevere. For the moment, though, let's consider more closely how the phrase "be made new in the attitude of your minds" works. Much of what we think about falls into three broad categories—people, ideas, and imaginings.

Learning to think in these areas in a godly manner is much the same as learning to act in a godly manner. Isolate a negative and decide what is its polar opposite. If envy is a problem, for example, decide what is its opposite. Acceptance? Contentment?

The three charts that follow may help clarify what we're talking about.

## How We Think about People

| OLD SELF | RENEWED MIND | NEW SELF |
|---|---|---|
| critical | God, help me | accepting |
| bitter | understand how | caring |
| resentful | you want me to | loving |
| envious | think about the | gracious |
| talking and com- | people in my life. | praying for people, |
| plaining about | | asking God to bless |
| people. | | and care for them. |

## How We Think about Ideas

| OLD SELF | RENEWED MIND | NEW SELF |
|---|---|---|
| If I do this, I'll get | How should I | I want to do what's |
| that. If I push hard | think about these | godly even if it's |
| enough, I'll get | hard issues, dear | not the easiest |
| what I want. After | Lord? Teach me | course to take. I |
| all, I deserve all I | your thoughts | must decrease and |
| can get. | and standards. | he must increase. |

## How We Think about Imaginings

| OLD SELF | RENEWED MIND | NEW SELF |
|---|---|---|
| I imagine myself | Lord, I want to | I imagine myself |
| rich, beautiful, sexy, | bring every | growing, sharing, |
| powerful, honored, | thought captive to | helping, encourag- |
| appreciated, with | Christ. | ing, loving, consis- |
| another man. | | tent—faithful. |

Suppose Tammy Boatwright had understood the full biblical equation for change. Suppose she had understood that she had to speak kindly to build her family up as well as she understood that she shouldn't speak nastily. Suppose she understood that she needed to learn to think as Christ thinks about the people she lives with. How might her morning have been different?

"Are you sick?" asked Hap when he saw her out of bed. "Don't you feel well?"

Automatically a defensive answer rose to her lips, but she knew she had to say something positive, not nasty.

"I feel fine," Tammy said. "I can't say morning's my favorite time, but I'll be okay."

Hap nodded in understanding as he climbed into the shower. "I'm not wild about mornings either."

Tammy smiled at herself as she brushed her teeth. Up five minutes and already she'd avoided an angry retort.

*Thanks, Lord.*

"By the way," yelled Hap over the roar of the water. "Do I have an ironed shirt for today?"

Tammy froze. An ironed shirt. She opened her mouth to say accusingly, "Why didn't you tell me yesterday that you were wearing your last one?" Instead she bit her lip. Such a response was at best a weak effort to transfer responsibility.

She peeked into the closet. No ironed shirt. She hurried to the laundry room. No ironed shirt. She sighed and looked in the washing machine. Lots of shirts, none ironed.

She pulled one out and threw it in the dryer. With any luck it would be done by the time Hap finished shaving.

Suddenly a loud and anguished "Mom!" pierced the air.

Tammy went flying to the rescue.

"He kicked me, Mom! He kicked me and knocked over my Lego building!" Alvin, her oldest, was standing in the middle of his room, pointing at the offender, two-year-old Darren.

Biting back a "Shut up, Alvin! You'll wake the dead!" Tammy said calmly, "Are you telling me that the baby kicked you so hard with his sleeper-covered feet that you're in great pain?"

"Yes," said Alvin. "I mean, no. I mean . . . "

Choosing not to say "Darren, you little animal, are you being a troublemaker again?" Tammy picked the baby up. "Come on, Sweetie; let's get some Cheerios. We want to leave Alvin alone so he can rebuild his beautiful building."

You may feel such a scenario sounds too easy to be true, and you may well be right. My point, though, is that when Tammy learned to make conscious choices by applying the entire put off/put on pattern, her quality of life improved dramatically.

By the grace of God, it can happen this way for all of us. It does take some meditation time; old patterns of viewing the world don't change quickly. You may need to ask repeatedly for the Holy Spirit to remind you what *God* thinks of people and situations, taking on a Christlike, *caring* attitude instead of the world's fault-finding and self-serving one.

You may even need to spend some time recreating discussions you've had (or imagining discussions you may have in the future), asking God's help in responding to others in an edifying fashion. (That's right—write yourself a script until it comes more naturally; *rehearse* kindness if you have to. How many times have you rehearsed biting remarks in your imagination?)

You may have to cut down on how much television you watch, because most sitcom dialogues teach us exactly how *not* to talk with one another; just count how many put-downs scriptwriters can fit into a minute's time. Have you noticed your kids sounding suspiciously similar to some of the obnoxious brats who appear regularly on screen in your family room?

We live in a me-first culture, and much of the verbal interchange between people day to day is not healthy. We push ahead in traffic, snarl at clerks (who sometimes snarl back more loudly), have a running inner commentary on what others wear, how they talk, even how they walk or move their hands in conversation. The only solution is to put on, put on, put on, the words and thoughts of our Lord, who was unselfish, concerned, empathetic, who looked at an out-of-sorts mob and "had compassion on them, for they were harrassed and helpless, like sheep without a shepherd." Jesus will give us radical thoughts, uplifting thoughts, thoughts and words that heal and reveal to people God's care for them and their worth to him.

## SUMMARY

Just recognizing what sinful things we want to change in our lives isn't enough.

The whole pattern of

1. putting off wrong things,
2. renewing our minds to agree with God about how we should do things, and
3. putting on the right or godly behavior is necessary to avoid a vacuum effect.

This put off/put on principle should apply to everything we think about—people, ideas, and imaginings—as well as to what we do.

## *What Do You Think?*

1. What habit or behavior has the Holy Spirit been convicting you about? If you put it off, what godly behavior should you put on in its place?


2. Read Colossians 3:5-10. What instructions are we given here? Why should we change?


3. Read Romans 12:2. What is the result of renewing your mind?


4. When Paul finished writing the examples of put off/put on in Ephesians 4, he wrote Ephesians 5:1-2. What two instructions has he for us as people with renewed minds?


5. In these same verses we see what putting on a life of love may require of us because of what it required of Christ. What is your response to such a cost?

# 10

# PERSEVERING PRACTICE

We have a black-and-white cat named Bugsy who thinks he's the world's greatest hunter. He loves to stalk squirrels and rabbits and birds. He refuses to let the fact that he has no foreclaws deter him. Instead he relies on speed and surprise.

Because he's a well-fed animal, Bugsy rarely shows an interest in eating his prey. His pleasure is mainly in the chase.

Many times I look out back and see him hiding behind a tree or a stump waiting for a gray squirrel to forget he's there. To my knowledge the squirrels have never been that foolish. If Bugsy does go for them, it's up a tree, just out of reach, they run. There they stop and deliver a loud and probably profane lecture.

While he has trouble with gray squirrels, Bugsy has reaped other prizes with his constant practice. I heard him "murp" one day and came to the door to find a baby rabbit cowering in a corner, completely unharmed but scared to death. I finally coaxed it to run into Chuck's slipper and, after carefully closing Bugsy inside, took the slipper and the rabbit to the woods and left them there. By the time Chuck came home, the rabbit was gone and the slipper back in the closet.

One night Bugsy brought in a flying squirrel still very much alive. I have no idea how he managed to catch it, but as soon as he loosened his hold on it, it began tearing around inside the house. We all watched and were properly impressed when it leaped off the top cellar step and flew down to the basement, rounding the bend in the steps very gracefully. Jeff was finally able to catch the little creature in a box and take him outside.

Unfortunately Jeff wasn't here last summer when Bugsy brought in a live chipmunk. Chuck and I tracked him to the back bedroom, then couldn't figure out how to get him out of there. He kept climbing up into the mechanism of the sofa-bed we keep there.

After several aborted and totally graceless tries, we finally got a box on top of him and slid a piece of stiff cardboard under him. We were barely out the back door when the cardboard separated from the box and the little guy was gone, hopefully never to return.

I am convinced that the main reason Bugsy has such success in spite of his lack of claws is because he practices and practices. For every success, there are many misses, many gray squirrel lectures. But if he didn't work so hard, he'd have all misses.

The same idea applies to developing emotional consistency. We need to practice, knowing there will be failures, but continuing to work at godly living until the successes are more frequent than the failures.

Anyone who lives on milk, being still an infant, is not acquainted with the teaching about righteousness. But solid food is for the mature, who by constant use have trained themselves to distinguish good from evil. *Hebrews 5:13-14*

# Practicing Godliness

I find it interesting that the writer of Hebrews says it is the mature believers who practice. It is the mature who by constant use have trained themselves to distinguish good from evil. It is the mature who persevere until they make the put off/put on pattern their way of living. It is the mature who recognize that renewing their minds is a spiritual skill that requires time and commitment.

God could have made us completely godly in our living patterns at the moment we trusted Christ. He could have. But as we all know from experience, he didn't. Instead he wants us to practice and grow and mature a step at a time. He wants us to persevere in being godly.

Perhaps it is a greater miracle than instant sanctification that in this world men and women choose to live holy lives simply because they love God and want to please him. Perhaps it is a greater miracle that they struggle against their natural tendencies, practicing, practicing, practicing godliness in order to be salt and light.

We're very used to the idea of athletes training hour after hour, performing a specific skill over and over when it doesn't count so that, when the competition finally does occur—when it finally does matter—they are prepared.

In the same way we as believers should be practicing, studying the Word, talking with the Lord, listening to those gifted in opening the Scriptures, making godly life choices in the small, daily things. Then, when the inevitable crunch comes, we will be ready to handle it in a manner that honors God.

When athletes train, they have their coaches to guide them and instruct them. The more gifted the coach, the better his athletes. The more teachable the athletes, the better their performances.

We have a Coach, too, who will guide and instruct us. The Holy Spirit delights in teaching us how to become more consistent. He rejoices in training us to be godly, in tutoring us to discern good from evil, in strengthening us for the trials ahead. It is our responsibility to be teachable, trainable believers.

As we commit our hearts to God and as the Holy Spirit leads us, we grow and we change. An acronym for "practice" will help us remember what's involved in these changes.

**P** rocess
**R** epetition
**A** ction
**C** ommitment
**T** edium
**I** ntegrity
**C** ommonality
**E** xcellence

## Process

When my boys were small, each summer we had membership to a pool in the area. The pool fielded a swimming team, and the boys wanted to be on it even though they couldn't get from one end of the pool to the other when they started and even though they had to practice every morning in the chilly air and water.

At one competition Jeff was chosen to swim the breast stroke in the eight-and-under category. I was delighted for him because he was so pleased. He took off as fast as he could and had the lead when one of the officials, walking down the side of the pool beside the racers, raised his fist and pointed to Jeff.

"DQ," the man said.

The child was disqualified because his kick was incorrect for the stroke. Somewhere along the line someone was supposed to teach the kids the proper kick, but it had never gotten done.

At the end of the meet when the eighteen-year-olds swam, it was another story. The training *process* and the year-in-and-year-out practice showed quite clearly.

Christian living is a *process*, too, not a static existence. Today we are not what we want to become, but we are also not what we were. We are advancing slowly, developing our own Christian histories, resting more on the Lord, learning step by step how to honor him. We are in process.

### Repetition

I am amazed at the discipline first-rate athletes have. They are willing to spend countless hours doing the same skill over and over, seeking a better swing, a greater body extension, a more fluid movement, or a fraction of a second off their time.

Christian living requires the discipline of *repetition*, too. Each day we commit ourselves to God. Each day we seek his will. Each day we make choices for his glory, not ours. Each day we say, "You must increase and I must decrease."

As an athlete cannot afford to grow careless about the basics, neither can we. When we rebel against *repetition*, we are in deep spiritual trouble.

### Action

After a life of having dogs as pets, I now have two cats. As I've compared them to the wonderful dogs in my past, I've concluded that they differ most dramatically from dogs in acting on command. Or, I should say, *not* acting on command.

Ask anything of a dog, and he'll try to make you happy, even if he hasn't the faintest idea what you want. He'll run in circles, bark, try to kiss you, or sit in your lap. A dog is an *action* animal.

A cat, on the other hand, will sit and stare at you no matter how elementary the command. He feels no need to please you, no need to act merely because you want him to.

While I hope that I would have a little more dignity than most dogs in my efforts to obey my Master's commands, I would hope I never develop a catlike hostility to action and practice. I want to say as Christ, "I have come to do your will, O God" (Hebrews 10:7).

## Commitment

There is one thing that our cats are committed to (besides eating), and that's protecting the sanctity of their home turf. A black-and-white cat has suddenly begun to visit us, and Bugsy and Fluffy are anything but pleased. In the cold weather when the sliding door was still closed, our guys would sit on the inside and this interloper would sit on the outside, and all three would howl and shriek and growl.

Now that the sliding door is open most of the day and evening and the cats are outside a lot, they are physically defending their territory. The other day I found Fluffy and this stranger locked in mortal combat with Bugsy running around making guttural noises.

I broke up the fight by touching Fluffy and the other cat on their backs and startling them so that they each let go. The strange cat took off with both my cats chasing him.

We believers don't wrestle (usually) with a physical enemy, as did our cats, but we certainly do engage daily, moment by moment, in spiritual warfare. We need to be absolutely *committed* to our God and to practicing holiness if we have any hope of being victorious.

## Tedium

I have noticed through the years that no matter what responsibility I have been given, and no matter how much I may enjoy that responsibility, part of the job has always been tedious. Keeping my files up to date and my desk clear are, to me, tedious chores. So are folding the wash and putting away the groceries. So are making the bed and preparing the garden for winter.

The Christian life is full of tedious moments, too. Cooking another meal for another new young mother, teaching Vacation Bible School for the 30 millionth year, preparing another Sunday school lesson for kids who rarely listen, washing up after a church dinner—after the first hundred times these jobs can lose their charm.

Christ probably found it tedious walking back and forth across Palestine under the hot Middle-Eastern sun, teaching the same thing over and over to people who didn't hear. Yet he did what he was supposed to do, *tedium* or no. So must we.

## Integrity

Several years ago when I flew home from a writers conference, my mom was to pick me up at the airport. I sat on a bench in the pick-up zone reading as I waited for her arrival. When she came I quickly tossed my things in her trunk.

We were getting out of the car at her house when I realized I didn't have my purse. I remembered setting it beside me on the bench, but I couldn't remember picking it up.

Mentally kissing my credit cards and money good-bye and dreading the complications of canceling everything and replacing it all, I went inside.

"Hi, Gayle. Lose something?" were my dad's first words.

A young woman had seen me get in Mom's car and drive off without my purse. She picked it up, took it home with her, and called to say she had it. Chuck and I stopped at her home in Philadelphia the next night to get the purse and thank her profusely.

Whenever I think of *integrity*, I think of this young woman. And I pray that I, as one who names the name of Christ, will be as honest and upright as she.

## Commonality

Many years ago I used to write a weekly column for our local paper. I would tell about the right-around-home things that happened in our family—Jeff's third birthday party, Chip's first-grade Halloween party with me as a homeroom mother, Chuck's pulled ligaments, my locking myself out in my bathrobe when no one was home. At the end of each column I'd have a spiritual parallel and a verse or a prayer.

I was completely surprised at the positive response to these little pieces. People even started asking Chuck, "Are you Gayle Roper's husband?" I especially loved this since we live in Chuck's hometown and people are always asking me which of the Ropers I'm related to.

The reason for the response to the columns was that I wrote about things all families experienced. My kids said funny things; their kids said funny things. I made a fool of myself; they made fools of themselves. *Commonality*.

There's *commonality* in our Christian experiences, too. As we practice godliness, we all struggle with establishing regular times with the Lord, with speaking only what encourages, with keeping the TV monster under control. And we all need the Lord's strength to keep on keeping on.

## Excellence

Several years ago when people first started asking me to autograph books I had written, I realized what an ego-inflater these requests were. It would be very easy to begin thinking that what I wrote was the last word in great writing.

I determined two things back then:

1. If what I wrote in a book or article was not based on the Word of God, it was no more than an opinion and as such could and should be readily ignored.
2. To remind myself where I must stand to have any real value to my readers, I began signing what has become my life verse, Colossians 3:17, after my name. "And whatever you do, whether in word or deed, do it all in the name of the Lord Jesus, giving thanks to God the Father through him."

As I practice doing everything in the name of Jesus, I have no choice but to strive for *excellence*. Anything less is simply not acceptable.

There is a song by Kelly Willard that spells out clearly what practice is all about and what it accomplishes.

*In a hidden valley just over the hill*
*A young shepherd boy surrenders his will*
*As he lifts his voice in praise to his King*
*Only the lambs will hear and follow as he sings.*

*Hidden valleys produce a life song*
*Hidden valleys will make a heart strong*
*Desperation can cause you to sing*
*Hidden valleys turn shepherds to kings.*

*In a hidden valley a faithful one leads*
*No one looking on, he cares for their needs*
*For he knows the One who tries the heart*
*So he is steadfast and content to do his part.*

*Hidden valleys produce a life song*
*Hidden valleys can make the heart strong*
*Desperation can cause us to sing*
*Hidden valleys turn shepherds to kings.*

*In a hidden valley a leader is born*
*He has faced the fierce and weathered the storm*
*So with humble heart and love for his God*
*He becomes royalty with just a staff and rod.*

*Hidden valleys produce a life song*
*Hidden valleys can make a heart strong*
*Desperation can cause you to sing*
*Hidden valleys turn shepherd to kings.*[1]

## SUMMARY

Practicing godly living over and over when no one's around trains us for the inevitable crunch.

We practice until there are more successes in godly living than failures.

God could have given us instant holiness when we became believers, but he chose to make us practice instead.

It's the practice, the hidden valleys, that turn us into kings.

## What Do You Think?

1. In his epistles Paul records his prayers for the various New Testament churches. What does he pray for believers and how does practice relate to these requests?

Ephesians 1:15-21

Ephesians 3:14-19

Philippians 1:9-11

Colossians 1:9-12

2. What area in your own Christian life needs practice? What plan of action will assist you as you practice?

3. Read Hebrews 6:12. How does this verse relate to practice?

# 11

# LEARNING CONTENTMENT

We were driving home from church one Sunday several years ago when Chip, then twelve going on twenty, asked, "Why do you always have to tell me what to do?"

I looked at my son, slouched so low that he was practically sitting on his neck.

"We all go to church, Chip. That's just one of the rules in our home."

"You don't have to make rules for me. I can take care of myself! I can't wait until I get out of this house!"

"You want to be free to go where you want when you want? To hang out with the kids you want? Go to bed when you want? Wear what you want? Stay home from church when you want?"

He seemed surprised that I understood. "That's it!"

I nodded. "As soon as you can pay your own rent, buy your own food, and afford the gas for your own car, you'll

113

be ready to be on your own. And of course there's washing your own clothes and paying to get yourself in wherever you want to go, too."

He looked at me, appalled.

"But," he said with all the sincerity and naivete of a kid, "I only want the good parts!"

I think many of us look at contentment as "the good parts." When we are at ease, when we are comfortable, when we have enough (whatever that is), we will be content. When life allows us to be as relaxed and fear-free and self-satisfied as a cat curled before a fire on a winter's night, then we will be content.

Scripturally, though, that definition doesn't work. It's much too American and land-of-plenty-ish. The Bible is a cross-cultural book. Any definitions for biblical concepts must apply in the poverty of Eastern Europe, the droughts of Saharan Africa and the cyclones of Bangladesh as well as the prosperity of the United States.

## Keys to Contentment

How, then, can believers with such different lives have a common understanding of contentment and the emotional consistency that comes with it?

### Sufficiency
To be content we must agree with God that he himself and what he has given us are sufficient for his purposes for us.

I don't understand how starvation fulfills God's purposes for some while garbage disposals full of leftovers satisfy his plan for others. I also don't know whether need or plenty is the greater block to people's turning to God.

I do know that if we strive for contentment, we won't find it. It's like happiness that way. It is a by-product of other things.

## *Obedience to God and his will*
To be content we must obey God no matter what the cost.

I don't understand why obedience has cost many believers so much through history while others of us pay so lightly for calling ourselves Christians. I also don't know whether imprisonment and martyrdom or acceptance and success are the greater blocks to people's living for Christ.

I do know that deep serenity and contentment are impossible when we are at war with God. We can fight this war on two fronts: pre-belief and post-belief.

Those who have not trusted Christ follow "the ways of this world and of the ruler of the kingdom of the air, the spirit who is now at work in those who are disobedient" (Ephesians 2:2). Unbelievers are often not aware that they are in combat with God and his people, but they are.

Believers, those who have trusted Christ and claimed his sacrificial death as the payment for their sins, can still rebel against their Father and his standards. One such example is found in Paul's words to the Corinthians, "You are still worldly. For since there is jealousy and quarreling among you, are you not worldly? Are you not acting like mere men?" (1 Corinthians 3:3).

When we obey God, the tension of our mutiny disappears and we are ready for the third key to contentment.

## *Learning*

I am not saying this because I am in need, for I have *learned to be content* whatever the circumstances. I know what it is to be in need, and I know what it is to have plenty. *I have learned the secret of being content* in any and every situation, whether well fed or hungry, whether living in plenty or in want. *Philippians 4:11-12, emphasis mine*

When Paul wrote this letter to the Philippians, he was a prisoner in Rome. When he wrote about being well-fed or hungry and living in plenty or in want, he wasn't exaggerating. He was admired and lauded on one hand and persecuted and hated on the other. Yet whatever the circumstances, he agreed with God that he had sufficient resources for God's purposes for him.

I first found Paul's thoughts on contentment in my teens, the traditional time for discontent. From then on these words have been a challenge to me in difficult situations.

When I was twenty-six and had a total hysterectomy and would never be able to have children, this verse challenged me to learn to be content with the unexpected path God had laid out for me.

When I entered a black period in my writing life where I went five years without a sale, again I prayed that I would learn to be content even if God's purpose for me was apparent failure.

When it became obvious that I was going to live the rest of my life with chronic back pain, I recalled Paul's "whatever the circumstances."

The fact that contentment is something to be learned reminds us again that the Christian life is a process. It's "precept upon precept, line upon line, here a little and there a little" (Isaiah 28:10, KJV).

### Farsightedness

To be satisfied with what God has provided for us, we have to see with eyes that look beyond today, eyes that look beyond our present problems. The promises of Christ's return and of heaven are given to us to foster this long view of things.

The New Testament is full of promises about the future because life for first-century Christians was so hard, so full of persecution. After his classic description of the Lord's return in 1 Thessalonians, Paul concludes, "Therefore encourage each other with these words" (4:18).

Now a man came up to Jesus and asked, "Teacher, what good thing must I do to get eternal life?"

"Why do you ask me about what is good?" Jesus replied. "There is only One who is good. If you want to enter life, obey the commandments."

"Which ones?" the man inquired.

Jesus replied, " 'Do not murder, do not commit adultery, do not steal, do not give false testimony, honor your father and mother,' and 'love your neighbor as yourself.' "

"All these I have kept," the young man said. "What do I still lack?"

Jesus answered, "If you want to be perfect, go, sell your possessions and give to the poor, and you will have treasure in heaven. Then come, follow me."

When the young man heard this, he went away sad, because he had great wealth. *Matthew 19:16-22*

This poor young man was unwilling to take the risks involved in finding contentment, and for him the risks were great. He had to give up his wealth, his lifestyle, his autonomy, his everything, and he was loath to do so.

He would not agree with Christ that God and his provision could be sufficient.

He would not be obedient to Christ's words.

He would not give himself any time to learn contentedness as Christ's follower.

And most of all, his vision of the *future* was completely colored by his *now*, by his wealth, by his own ideas of what was best for him.

Doesn't he sound just like us?

I confess that farsightedness is the most difficult part of contentment for me. I have a hard time working up great enthusiasm for being with the Lord either by his coming or by my going. My life is too pleasant.

I look out my back door at the lushness of my flower garden with its marvelous shades of ruby, sapphire, fuchsia and emerald, and I like it right here.

I lie in my warm, dry bed and listen to the rain pelt the roof and tumble down the drain, and I like it here.

I watch my sons become fine young men, I hold my granddaughter Ashley on my lap and read to her, I enjoy a dinner out with Chuck, and I like it here.

While in one sense God has blessed me as "the lines have fallen to me in pleasant places," in another sense I have lost the edge of appreciating God's future for me. I have more in common with the rich young ruler than I like to admit.

## SUMMARY

Contentment is agreeing with God that he and his provision for us are sufficient for his purposes for us.

Obeying God is a prerequisite for contentment.

Contentment is something we can learn whatever our circumstances.

A contented Christian is far-sighted, loving the promises of Christ's return and of heaven.

## *What Do You Think?*

1. Is there an area in your life where you find yourself disagreeing with God about his provision for you? Or his provision for someone else?

2. *Webster's New World Dictionary* defines contentment as being satisfied. From a natural, human point of view, is contentment possible? How does a Christian's understanding of contentment differ from the world's?

3. Read Proverbs 19:23. What is necessary before a person can "rest content"?

4. Can contentment and ambition coexist? Contentment and progress? Contentment and dreams and goals? Is contentment the same thing as complacency?

5. Read 1 Timothy 6:6-10. How does this passage remind you of the rich young ruler? What lessons are especially pertinent to you?

# 12

# ROOTED COMMITMENT

Aha! I finally knew what I would do for my four sisters-in-law for Christmas. I'd give each of them a bulb garden that would bloom in January and February. Then every time they looked at or smelled the narcissus, they would think, *How clever and kind of Gayle to give such a thoughtful gift.*

At least I knew that's what I'd think if I got a gift that nice.

I ordered the bulbs from one of the best mail-order gardening supply companies. I carefully read all that I could find on how to create and raise healthy bulb gardens. I bought the soil recommended and the pots to contain these marvelous gifts.

I planted the bulbs in November as advised, taking care that they were placed at just the right depth in the pots. I put them in the garage, which was both dark and cool. I watered them only as much as I was told. And I waited.

The pots I had gotten were clear plastic, and when I'd check on the progress of my gardens, I could see the root systems developing. I was fascinated by the hairy white

tendrils pushing their way through the soil, and I was confident I'd have a superior product to give. When tiny sprouts
appeared on the bulbs, I knew all was in good order.

Then I noticed that the little sprouts weren't growing
taller, and their color was no longer a healthy, pliant green.
Soon they were a crisp, very dead brown.

Somehow, and I still don't know exactly how, I'd killed
my wonderful gifts. The week before Christmas I was out
frantically looking for something else to give my sisters-in-
law.

Now for my analogy. After all, I must get some value out
of those dead plants.

> So then, just as you received Christ Jesus as Lord, continue
> to live in him, *rooted* and built up in him, strengthened in
> the faith as you were taught, and overflowing with
> thankfulness. *Colossians 2:6-7, emphasis mine*

## Rooted in Christ

When I think of what our relationship with Christ is to be, I
think of those wonderful root systems my bulbs developed.
I can see in my mind's eye the young shoots growing down
into that soil and burying themselves in it, drawing life
from it.

That's the way we need to bury ourselves in Christ, rooting ourselves firmly in him. As a strong root system
anchors a plant in the ground, protecting it from winds and
storms, so burrowing deep in Christ protects us from the
potential ravages of life's storms.

A good root system also provides nourishment to a plant,
pulling water and chemicals from the soil and through

capillary action passing these life-giving necessities to the entire plant.

Similarly our roots buried deep in Christ, the Bread of Life and the Living Water, nourish us, enabling us to grow and to blossom in the most extraordinarily difficult circumstances as well as in the pleasant, sunny places.

My analogy breaks down at this point as all analogies eventually must. My bulb gardens never grew due to the limitations of their gardener. But we have the Master Gardener tending us, and he knows exactly how to care for us, how to encourage us, how to rescue us.

This is what the LORD says: "Cursed is the one who trusts in man, who depends on flesh for his strength and whose heart turns away from the LORD. He will be like a bush in the wastelands; he will not see prosperity when it comes. He will dwell in the parched places of the desert, in a salt land where no one lives.

"But blessed is the man who trusts in the LORD, whose confidence is in him. He will be like a tree planted by the water that sends out its roots by the stream. It does not fear when heat comes; its leaves are always green. It has no worries in a year of drought and never fails to bear fruit." *Jeremiah 17:5-8*

What about us? Will we be a bush in the wastelands, depending on our own strength? Or will we be a tree planted by the water, our confidence in God?

When we ask that question cloaked in the illustration of bushes in wastelands and trees strong by the stream, the answer seems so obvious. None of us wants to be a bush in a wasteland. We all want to prosper and grow.

However, asked straight out, stripped of all picturesque language, the question is harder to answer.

*Are we willing to be so rooted in Christ that we trust only in him, choosing always to do his will, opting always to follow his lead, deciding always to yield our todays and tomorrows to him?*

## Core Issue

The question of commitment, of becoming wholly God's woman, is the core issue of learning to be emotionally consistent. It is from this basic decision that all our godly options flow.

We can learn how to set godly and reachable goals when we become willing to do it his way instead of ours.

We understand that God values us and will use us no matter how self-confident we may or may not be when we say, "Lord, I'm yours."

We learn how to enjoy our emotions and develop our thoughts when we follow the example of Christ in the Garden.

We are able to develop strong, godly patterns when we say, "Lord, I'm not only willing to do it your way. I *want* to do it your way."

We learn to deal with real and assumed guilt when we depend fully on Christ, the Forgiver of sins and the Bearer of burdens.

Now I have another question for us all. If commitment is what God asks of us and if it is so profitable for ordering our lives, why don't we immediately and easily give God our all?

There are several possible answers to this question, ranging from a rebellious spirit to fear, from the captain-of-my-fate and master-of-my-soul syndrome to peer pressure. I'd like us to look at the cares of life and the "dailiness" of living as major culprits that mitigate against commitment.

## The Major Culprits

It's not that we don't love God. We do. We talk to him whenever we have time. It's just that time is so limited and there are so many other things, so many good things that must be done. We're caught in the tyranny of the urgent.

It's not that we're angry with God or overtly rebellious. We think God's principles as presented in the Bible are very wise and practical. It's just that applying these principles takes more concentration and energy than we have or are willing to expend.

And it's not that we don't recognize pain all about us. We most certainly do, and we agree that the church should be getting involved in needy lives with the healing message of salvation and commitment. It's just that our present priorities are our families and our jobs. When these situations ease up, then we'll think seriously about all that God asks of us.

Do these thought patterns sound familiar? They are ages old. We're certainly not the first ones to be distracted from our highest goal by merely important goals.

King Solomon, however, loved many foreign women besides Pharaoh's daughter—Moabites, Ammonites, Edomites, Sidonians and Hittites. They were from nations about which the LORD had told the Israelites, "You must not intermarry with them, because they will surely turn your hearts after their gods."

Nevertheless, Solomon held fast to them in love. He had seven hundred wives of royal birth and three

hundred concubines, and his wives led him astray. As Solomon grew old, his wives turned his heart after other gods, and his heart was not fully devoted to the LORD his God, as the heart of David his father had been. He followed Ashtoreth the goddess of the Sidonians, and Molech the detestable god of the Ammonites. So Solomon did evil in the eyes of the LORD; he did not follow the LORD completely, as David his father had done.
*1 Kings 11:1-6*

Many of Solomon's wives and concubines were acquired because it was politically expedient for him to have links with the surrounding nations as a means of keeping peace in the region. Certainly a great and wealthy king like Solomon could convince himself that peace was primary, and if keeping it meant bending the laws of God concerning intermarriage with godless nations, well, so be it. God would understand.

Of course, once Solomon had all these women, he was responsible for their care and for the care of his children by them. Apparently one way he showed his concern for them—and one way he kept peace in the seraglio, I imagine—was to allow these foreign women to keep their gods. Again expedience led Solomon to disregard another of God's absolute commands, this one to keep Israel clean of idols.

For the wisest man who ever lived, Solomon had a remarkable ability to deceive himself.

Solomon's most serious step away from God, the God he still claimed to love and the God who allowed him to build the temple in spite of his sin, was when the influence of his foreign wives led him to worship their gods, even the loathsome god Molech to whom child sacrifices were offered.

Solomon's commitment to God was undermined by the "dailiness" and expedience of his life. His choices meant "his heart was not fully devoted to the Lord his God" and "he did not follow the Lord completely."

Granted, we don't normally make decisions on the scale of Solomon, but our choices will influence our lives every bit as strongly as Solomon's heathen wives impacted his.

I know that when I die, I do NOT want people to speak of me as Scripture does of Solomon: "His heart was not fully devoted to the Lord his God." Rather I want to be known, as Paul was, as a servant of God who could write, "I have fought the good fight, I have finished the race, I have kept the faith" (2 Timothy 4:7).

*God, we all want emotional consistency and control. The cost of realizing these things is everything and nothing—everything as we know our lives and nothing compared to the benefits and blessings you will give us. May we in our commitment to you be a sweet fragrance to you and to the world around us. Amen.*

## SUMMARY

Commitment is rooting ourselves in Christ as our Anchor and our Provider.

Total commitment to God is at the core of emotional consistency.

The "dailiness" of life can undercut our commitment to God. Solomon is an example of this occurrence.

## What Do You Think?

1. We have talked about digging our roots deep in Christ. Read Hebrews 12:15 and Deuteronomy 29:18. What do these verses warn about roots?

2. The parable of the sower mentions the importance of roots. Read Matthew 13:21-22. What does it teach us about roots?

3. When you think about committing your life to Christ completely, what gives you greatest concern or hesitation?

4. Read Romans 14:8. How does the eternal perspective in this verse help you in thinking about commitment?

5. Read Philippians 3:7-10. How does Paul explain the depths of his commitment to Christ?